Equine Bandaging, Splinting,
and Casting Techniques

Equine Bandaging, Splinting, and Casting Techniques

J Dylan Lutter, Haileigh Avellar, and Jen Panzer

Equine Surgery
Department of Clinical Sciences
Veterinary Health Center
College of Veterinary Medicine
Kansas State University
Manhattan, KS, US

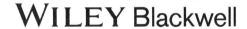

Published by John Wiley & Sons, Inc., Hoboken, New Jersey.
Published simultaneously in Canada.

For general information on our other products and services or for technical support, please contact our
Customer Care Department within the United States at (800) 762-2974, outside the United States at
(317) 572-3993 or fax (317) 572-4002.

Wiley also publishes its books in a variety of electronic formats. Some content that appears in print may
not be available in electronic formats. For more information about Wiley products, visit our web site at
www.wiley.com.

Library of Congress Cataloging-in-Publication Data
Names: Lutter, J Dylan, 1982– author. | Avellar, Haileigh, author.
  | Panzer, Jen, author.
Title: Equine bandaging, splinting, and casting techniques / J Dylan
  Lutter, Haileigh Avellar, Jen Panzer.
Description: Hoboken, New Jersey : Wiley Blackwell, [2024] | Includes
  index.
Identifiers: LCCN 2024000512 (print) | LCCN 2024000513 (ebook) | ISBN
  9781119841838 (paperback) | ISBN 9781119841852 (adobe pdf) | ISBN
  9781119841845 (epub)
Subjects: MESH: Horse Diseases–surgery | Fracture Fixation–veterinary |
  Extremities–injuries | Bandages–veterinary | Splints–veterinary |
  Casts, Surgical–veterinary
Classification: LCC SF959.F78 (print) | LCC SF959.F78 (ebook) | NLM SF
  959.F78 | DDC 636.1/089705–dc23/eng/20240202
LC record available at https://lccn.loc.gov/2024000512
LC ebook record available at https://lccn.loc.gov/2024000513

Cover Design: Wiley
Cover Image: Courtesy of J Dylan Lutter

Set in 9.5/12.5pt STIXTwoText by Straive, Pondicherry, India
SKY10068706_030124

Contents

Preface

I (JDL) first became interested in equine bandaging during my residency with the small project I published that qualified me to take the American College of Veterinary Surgeons' board exam. That project showed me how few resources there are in veterinary medicine about bandaging and more specifically the splinting of equine fractures. The majority of the articles written are review articles in which the authors state their personal experiences and reference the experiences of previous authors who have written other review articles or textbook chapters. At the time, there were no objective studies evaluating the effectiveness of the most commonly recommended fracture splinting techniques and very few studies investigating the effects of various bandaging techniques. There were also no available books dedicated to teaching the methods of bandaging, splinting, and casting equine limbs. Nearly all of the techniques used in these areas are passed down from person to person, each putting their own preferences and nuances onto those methods.

The purpose of this book is to address some of these deficiencies by providing step-by-step images with thorough descriptions of each step. It is not intended to be a reference text. Instead, it is written as a practical handbook that presents the authors' approach to equine bandaging, splinting, and casting.

About the Companion Website

This book is accompanied by a companion website.

www.wiley.com/go/lutter/1e

This website includes:

- Figure PPTs

Section I

Application of Equine Bandages

1

Materials and Concepts for Bandage Application

Bandages are frequently applied in equine veterinary medicine and are useful for a variety of purposes. Most commonly, bandages are applied to protect and manage the environment of a wound or surgical site while healing commences. At other times they are applied to help control/prevent edema, to provide compression and physical support to injured tissues, or to reduce the motion of a limb or region. A thorough discussion of the indications for and benefits of a bandage are well discussed elsewhere (see Suggested Reading at the end of this chapter) and are beyond the scope of this book. Suffice it to say that a properly applied bandage is generally beneficial to wound healing and greatly aids in the management of numerous equine disorders, but an inappropriately applied bandage may do far more harm than the issue for which that bandage was applied.

Bandage Layers

A bandage is composed of primary, secondary, and tertiary layers. Each of these layers serves a specific purpose and may be composed of a single kind or multiple types of material. In some instances a single material may serve the purpose of more than one layer. It is up to each clinician to evaluate the patient and the reasons for bandage application in order to determine which materials to use. In most cases a standard list of materials will be used, but in certain circumstances a material may be omitted, substituted, or added for a specific purpose. Additionally, the "standard bandage" will vary by where the veterinary practice is located, by practice type, client expectations, clinician preferences, and even by tradition. The bandage techniques shown in this book will represent one version of the "standard bandage" that can be broadly adopted regardless of these variables.

Equine Bandaging, Splinting, and Casting Techniques, First Edition. J Dylan Lutter, Haileigh Avellar, and Jen Panzer.
© 2024 John Wiley & Sons, Inc. Published 2024 by John Wiley & Sons, Inc.
Companion website: www.wiley.com/go/lutter/1e

Primary Layer

The primary layer of a bandage is otherwise known as the contact layer or the wound dressing. The material applied in this layer directly interacts with the skin or wound below it. It may be used to deliver a medication, absorb exudate, debride tissue, or provide a sealed barrier. The most common material used as a primary layer in equine bandages is a telfa pad, which is classified as a non-adherent, non-occlusive, mildly absorptive wound dressing (Figure 1.1). Table 1.1 lists some commonly used dressings and their classifications. The effect of these dressings is more appropriate in a discussion of wound management and will not be further covered here.

Secondary Layer

The secondary layer is typically composed of a soft, conformable, compressible, and absorptive material (Figure 1.2). In wound management, this layer acts to absorb moisture (sweat) and wound exudate and creates a continuous barrier between the underlying tissue and the external environment while also holding any wound dressings in place. The secondary layer also reduces the contours of the limb, making it more cylindrical, and acts as a cushion to the limb due to its compressible nature. Both of these properties protect the underlying limb from

(a)   (b)

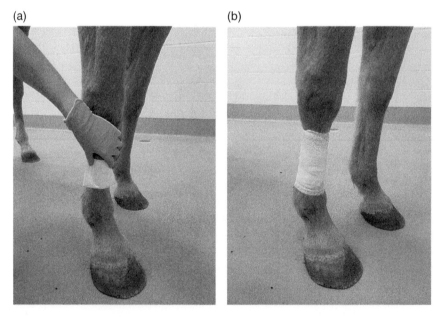

Figure 1.1   A telfa pad is a wound dressing commonly used as a primary layer of a bandage. It should be large enough to cover the wound and may either be (a) held in place with the bandager's hand while the secondary bandage layer is applied or (b) secured to the limb using inelastic woven gauze applied with no tension.

Table 1.1 Commonly used wound dressings and their classification.

Dressing type	Use
Gauze	Exudate absorption; superficial debridement if applied without a non-adherent covering
Alginate	Exudate absorption; promotion of hemostatic, inflammatory, autolytic debridement, and proliferative stages of wound healing
Cellulose/hydrofiber	Promotion of moist wound healing/granulation; similar to alginate but not for use in bleeding wounds
Chitin/chitosan	For control of hemorrhage following initial wound occurrence
Hydrogel	Used in clean acute wounds that are non-exudative/dry to promote autolytic wound debridement and initial moist wound healing; not for infected wounds
Hydrocolloid	Used in clean acute wounds during the inflammatory and early proliferative phases of wound healing; not for infected wounds
Foam	Exudate absorption and wound moisture maintenance in exudative wounds once the wound is filled with granulation tissue; promotes epithelization and wound contraction
Silicone	Fully occlusive wound dressing used to control and prevent occurrence of exuberant granulation tissue

(a) (b)

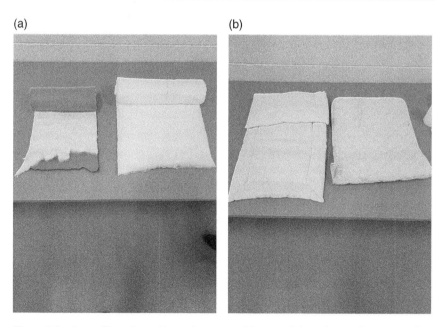

Figure 1.2 Any soft, conformable, and compressible material can be used as a secondary layer of bandage. (a) Disposable materials such as loose roll cotton or CombiRoll® are convenient and commonly used when dealing with wounds that can thoroughly soil a bandage. (b) Reusable materials such as the bandage quilts shown or even soft towels can be used to reduce costs, but may be difficult to clean or become damaged before the cost is recouped.

Table 1.2 Commonly used materials for the secondary layer bandage.

Material	Use/function
Conform gauze	Woven gauze of various widths used to secure the wound dressing
Cotton cast padding	Easily torn thin sheet of cotton used in bandages to secure the wound dressing
Unlined cotton roll	Thick, compressible sheets of loose cotton that may be applied for bandage padding and exudate absorption. Easily torn and potentially messy to use, as cotton fibers may adhere to the wound
Lined cotton roll	Most commonly used material for the secondary bandage layer. Cotton roll with a thin cotton lining surrounding it to contain the cotton and provide additional strength/structure to the material
Quilt wrap	Washable cotton fabric containing a cushion layer that is washable and reusable

external forces that may be applied to it. Most importantly, this layer protects and effectively distributes the forces applied to the limb by the tensioned materials of the tertiary bandage layer.

Conveniently, in equine practice a disposable cotton roll is commonly used. Other disposable items such as rolled gauze or cotton cast padding may be used if absorption is of little importance or if little to no tension will be applied to the tertiary layers. Non-disposable items such as quilt wraps or even towels and cut blankets may be substituted in an emergency (Table 1.2).

Tertiary Layer

The tertiary layer of a bandage is typically composed of one or two different types of materials and has a primary purpose of providing compression (Figure 1.3). The first material applied after the secondary layer should be an inelastic, woven gauze. This inner tertiary layer provides most of the compression of the underlying bandage materials, holding the bandage together and helping to stiffen it. The second outer material is typically an extensible material that, when tension is applied to it, further compresses the underlying bandage materials and stiffens the bandage. The outer tertiary bandage material should be sturdier than the materials in the underlying layers and frequently has water-resistant properties. Both of these characteristics add an environmental protection component to the purposes of this bandage layer. Most frequently elastic, cohesive bandage materials are used as the outer tertiary bandage layer (Figure 1.4).

On occasion, a clinician may choose to omit either the inner gauze material or the outer cohesive material of the tertiary layer. This is often done as a cost-saving measure. However, in doing so the clinician must be aware of the trade-offs and decide if it is worth the risk. These trade-offs include reduced compression of the

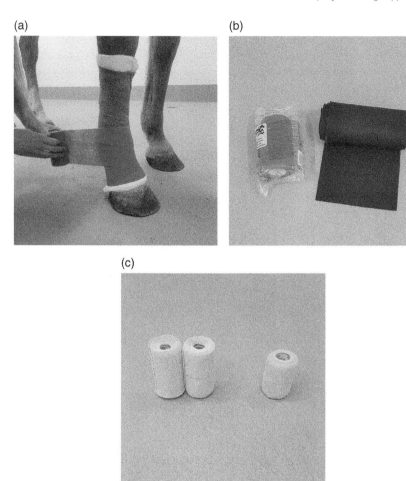

Figure 1.3 The tertiary layer of a bandage may be composed of either one or multiple different materials used in various combinations to add compression and stiffness to the bandage. (a) A standard bandage is shown using cohesive bandage material and woven brown gauze. (b) A polo wrap can be used to reduce bandage material waste, but can be less effective at staying in place and may need to be replaced more frequently. (c) If further compression or bandage stiffness is desired, additional material, such as elastic adhesive bandage (shown) or another cohesive bandage, may be applied on top of the standard cohesive bandage/brown gauze layer. The added benefit of these additional layers diminishes with each subsequent layer.

bandage material, a less stiff/sturdy bandage, reduced support to the underlying anatomy, and (in the case of omitting cohesive material) reduced environmental protection. Table 1.3 contains a partial list of the available materials used for the tertiary layer. Elastic non-cohesive bandage materials, such as an ACE™ bandage or a "polo" wrap, can be used with or without brown gauze as the tertiary bandage

(a) (b)

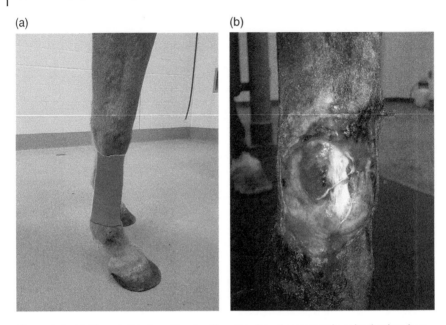

Figure 1.4 (a) Though it is tempting to allow this for minor wounds, cohesive bandage material should never contact skin. (b) It may constrict over time, restrict blood flow, and cause tissue damage or even skin sloughing.

Table 1.3 Commonly used materials for the tertiary layer bandage.

Material	Use/function
Woven brown gauze	Inelastic, easily torn woven gauze used immediately after the secondary padding layer to compress the padding and conform it to the leg
Cohesive bandage	Elastic self-adherent conforming material used to compress the secondary bandage material layer, conform it to the leg, and provide a semi-water-resistant protective layer. May include latex or be latex free, and may come with adhesive glue applied. Should not be applied directly to skin
Adhesive elastic tape	Woven fabric tape with adhesive applied to secure and seal the ends of a bandage. Should only be applied to skin without applying tension
Polo wrap	Commonly used supportive leg wrap in the equine industry. May be used as a washable alternative to the cohesive bandage to compress and secure the secondary bandage layer. Typically does not result in as secure a bandage as the cohesive bandage

layer. Because they are reusable they can provide a measure of cost saving, especially in cases where bandages are required for many days or weeks. However, these materials do not provide the same measure of bandage stiffness/sturdiness and environmental protection as a cohesive bandage material.

Elastic adhesive bandage tape may also be used as the tertiary bandage layer, especially in cases where the extra adhesion of the material to the underlying layers and to itself is desired to produce a sturdier bandage. The major downsides of using this material include the cost of the elastic bandage tape and its absorptive/woven nature, which provides a lower degree of environmental contamination protection. Occasionally, some clinicians may choose to apply a layer of cohesive bandage followed by a layer of adhesive bandage. Finally, regardless of the type of material chosen for the tertiary bandage layer, the ends of the bandage are frequently sealed using elastic tape applied without tension to prevent the migration of dirt and debris inside the bandage.

Additional Protection of the Bandage

In some cases, additional materials or techniques need to be employed to protect the bandage itself from damage, environmental contamination, or moisture. Table 1.4 lists some problems that commonly present and some possible solutions.

Table 1.4 Problems that may occur causing excessive damage, soiling, or moisture to a horse's bandage, along with some possible solutions.

Problem	Solution
A horse that needs a bath or cold hydrotherapy (i.e. cold-hosing) while the bandage remains in place	Tape a plastic barrier over the bandage (rectal sleeve, trash bag)
A horse with excessive purulent drainage or diarrhea	Tape a plastic barrier over the bandage or apply a water repellent (petrolatum jelly)
A horse housed in an excessively dirty or moist environment (i.e. if a stall is not available at a client's home)	Tape a plastic barrier over the bandage; plan to change the bandage more frequently
A horse that chews the bandage or is attempting to self-mutilate	Apply a chew deterrent – cayenne pepper mixed with petrolatum jelly is highly effective, or apply additional layers to the bandage such as elastic adhesive bandage tape or even duct tape
A horse excessively rubbing the bandage	Apply additional layers of tougher bandage material. Elastic adhesive tape may be effective, but also has a high coefficient of friction so it may make matters worse. The authors have found that applying slippery tape such as duct tape in a vertical fashion to the high-rub areas and (if needed) topping it with petrolatum jelly is effective in some cases

Application of Bandage Materials

Proper application of the bandage materials is as important, if not more important, than the bandage materials themselves. Inappropriate application of even the best bandage materials will, at best, result in a bandage that needs to be more frequently changed and, at worst, result in complete bandage failure with subsequent destruction of the surgical site or wound repair.

Order of Application

In general, the only materials allowed to touch the skin of the animal should be wound dressing/conforming gauze (aka the primary bandage layer) and the inner surface of the absorptive/compressible secondary bandage layer.

Cohesive bandage material should never be applied circumferentially directly to the skin (Figure 1.4). If this is done and the bandage material constricts or swelling occurs, the blood supply to the area will be disrupted. If allowed to continue long enough a bandage sore, skin sloughing, or even hoof sloughing will develop. These materials should only be applied on top of sufficient padding to protect the underlying anatomy. There are two exceptions to this rule. The first is the application of elastic adhesive bandage tape directly to the skin *without* tension, either as an inner protective layer or to seal the ends of a complete bandage (Figure 1.5). Even this carries some risk that the bandage tape will slip, bunch up, and potentially cause constriction. The second exception is the use of a non-circumferential piece of tape to hold some material in place.

Amount of Padding

The amount of padding used in the secondary bandage layer may vary with each individual situation. The "correct" amount to be used should follow the Goldilocks approach: not too little and not too much but just enough. In general, it is better to err on the side of a little more padding to ensure adequate protection of the limb. Pre-cut and rolled material can be purchased that is cut to an adequate length, but bulk cotton combine can be purchased in 10 m rolls and cut to any desired length. The authors find that a length of 50–55 cm is a good length to fit many different applications and will easily wrap around the limb 1.5–2 times.

Tension

The amount of tension applied during bandage application will vary depending on which layer of bandage is being applied, the anatomic location being bandaged, and the purpose of the bandage. The primary bandage layer should always

(a)

(b)

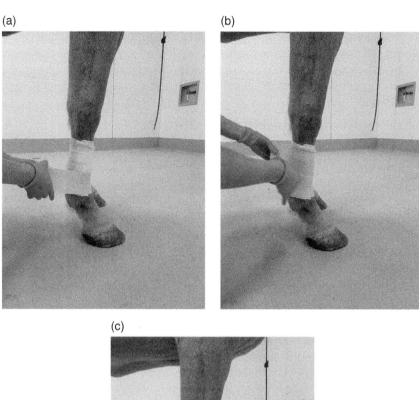

(c)

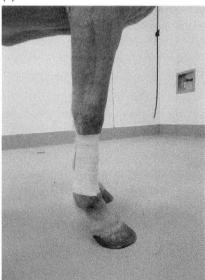

Figure 1.5 (a–c) If added security of the primary bandage layer is desired to either protect a surgical site from contamination or to protect the skin from damage, then elastic adhesive bandage material, *applied without tension*, may be added to the bandage. It is important that no tension is applied to this material to avoid restriction of blood flow to the limb and potential tissue damage.

be applied without tension to avoid the potential for material constriction. Tension is not required to apply the secondary bandage layer, as this layer will be compressed and held in place by the tertiary layer. However, applying the secondary layer so that it is neatly arranged, not bunched up, and will not spin around the limb will generally improve the quality and appearance of the bandage. Tension applied to the tertiary layer will vary, but should be sufficient to compress the underlying layers and hold the bandage material together.

- The most important concept is that the tertiary layer should be applied with even tension for the entire length of the bandage.

If uneven tension is applied, whereby one wrap is taken very tightly followed by a loose wrap and then another tight wrap, the forces applied to the limb will concentrate at these areas of uneven tension and damage the tissues in those areas (Figure 1.6). At best, this will result in unnecessary edema and inflammation in the area. At worst, it will result in pressure necrosis of the affected tissues due to disrupted blood supply or in the creation of tendon/ligament injury under the bandage (commonly known in the equine industry as a "bandage bow," as in a "bowed tendon").

Because the equine distal limb contains little soft tissue compared to small animal patients, the amount of tension that can be applied to equine limb bandages is substantially higher than in small animals. In horses, both the inner and outer tertiary bandage materials could be applied with enough tension to the point of ripping without damaging the limb, provided that sufficient padding is used and even tension is applied for the entire bandage.

- A balance must be achieved through practice and experience in order to produce a bandage that is safe for the horse, yet stiff enough to achieve the purpose of the bandage and prevent the need for excessive bandage changes.

The more loosely a bandage is applied, the lower the risk of bandage-related injury but the higher the likelihood of an insufficient bandage. A tightly applied bandage will be more structurally sound and provide more support to the underlying limb than a loose bandage. However, the more tightly a bandage is applied, the higher the risk of applying uneven tension and thus the higher the risk of bandage-related injury.

Six-inch-wide woven brown gauze is nearly universally used by veterinarians as the inner tertiary layer in equine bandages. It should be applied with sufficient tension to compress the underlying bandage material and hold the bandage together. This material can be easily ripped if excessive tension is applied to it and it is nearly impossible to apply it too tightly, *as long as even tension is applied for the entire bandage.* Four-inch-wide cohesive bandage is the preferred outer tertiary bandage material. This should be applied with enough tension to further

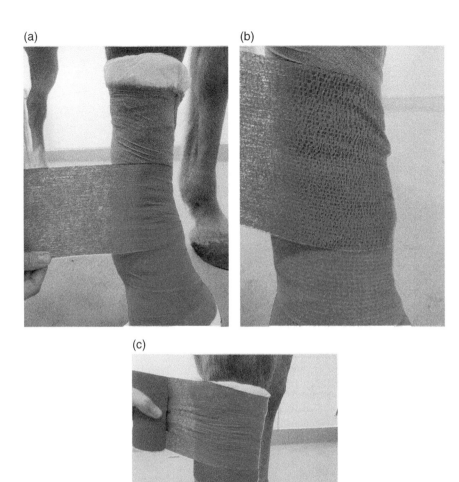

Figure 1.6 The tertiary bandage layer must be applied with appropriate tension to construct a quality bandage. (a) The cohesive bandage material shown is being stretched sufficiently, which eliminates the elastic "crinkles" in the material. (b) The cohesive bandage material shown here is not being stretched sufficiently and the "crinkles" are easily visible. A bandage applied with this tension will not provide sufficient support to the limb and will not hold together as well as a bandage applied with appropriate tension. (c) It is important to apply the bandage material with even tension. Shown is an area of loosely applied material surrounded by an area of tightly applied material. The loose area will concentrate bandaging forces and predispose to the development of tissue damage, such as a bandage bow.

compress the underlying materials and allow the cohesive bandage material to stick to itself and form a uniform outer layer.

- A good guideline is to apply enough tension to the cohesive bandage material so that the crinkles are removed, resulting in a smooth appearance.

For typical bandages this cohesive material is not stretched to the point of ripping. As will be discussed in the splinting chapters, a substantial amount of additional tensile force can be applied after the crinkles disappear to further increase the overall bandage stiffness.

- If a bandage has been well applied, with sufficient tension to all layers (aka a good tight bandage), it will sound like a ripe melon when flicked with your finger.

Wrapping the Material

When applying the bandage to the limb, the specific details of wrapping the material become important to create a good-quality bandage and to make the bandage application process as efficient as possible. One detail that is frequently considered and debated is the direction in which the bandage material should be wrapped (Figure 1.7).

(a)   (b)

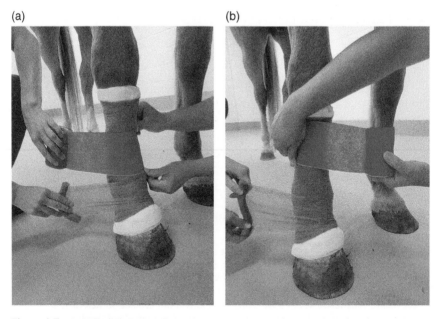

Figure 1.7 (a, b) Each bandage layer should be wrapped in the same direction. Switching directions between layers will counteract some of the tension applied and result in a less effective bandage.

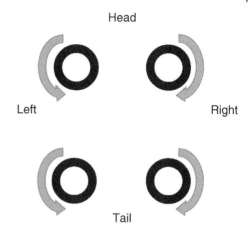

Figure 1.8 Despite there being no medical reason for it, the industry-accepted direction of wrapping the bandage material is to "wrap the tendons in." When viewed from above, the left limbs will be wrapped in a counterclockwise direction and the right limbs will be wrapped in a clockwise direction.

The standard "correct way" in the horse industry is to "wrap the tendons in" (Figure 1.8). This standard way to wrap is based largely on tradition and dogma. The idea is that wrapping the flexor tendons "in" (i.e. medially) somehow protects them from injury, but it has no scientific basis to back it up.

From a medical standpoint, it makes no difference which direction the bandage material is wrapped. However, veterinarians continue to conform to the industry standard direction, primarily to avoid controversy and conflict with some owners and trainers.

The conventional way to wrap also begs the question of "Which way is in?" More accurately stated, if the horse is viewed from above, the right limbs should be wrapped in a clockwise direction and the left limbs should be wrapped in a counterclockwise direction. On an anatomic basis, the bandage material should pass on the lateral aspect of the limb from dorsal to palmar/plantar and then medially. Both descriptions are somewhat cumbersome to explain, so hopefully the reader can appreciate why the standard phrase has become to "wrap the tendons in." When wrapping, the roll of material should be placed so that it unrolls onto the leg instead of unrolling away from the leg. Figure 1.9 illustrates this concept.

Another area where dogma exists within the equine industry is regarding where to start wrapping (i.e. top, middle, or bottom of the bandage). From a practical standpoint, it makes no difference where one starts. One of the authors (JDL) prefers to start at the top of the bandage because he feels it helps him hold all of the materials together neatly when bandaging without assistance. He progresses to wrap distally and then return proximally until the material runs out. Other individuals prefer always to start their tertiary layers in the middle of the bandage and wrap either distally or proximally as the situation dictates. Starting at the bottom of the bandage may make logical sense if the bandager is trying to

(a)   (b)

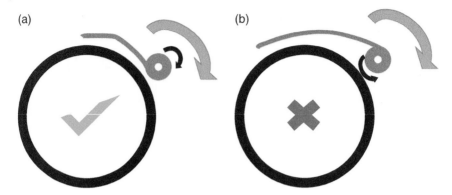

Figure 1.9 (a) When applying bandage material to the leg, the roll of material should be held so that it unrolls onto the leg. Incidentally, this will coincide with the direction of wrapping around the leg. (b) Conversely, if the roll of material is held so that it unrolls away from the leg (i.e. opposite to the direction of wrapping), the bandage application will be more cumbersome and prone to error.

squeeze edema or fluid proximally out of the limb. While no scientific evidence of this exists in horses, studies are being undertaken to investigate the occurrence and potential benefit of the approach. Regardless of where the tertiary wraps are started, it is important to leave approximately one finger's width of cotton showing at the top and bottom of the bandage. This ensures there is sufficient padding in place to protect the limb from the tension being applied to the tertiary layer.

As the tertiary bandage materials (brown gauze and cohesive bandage) are being applied, the material should be wrapped once around the limb to bind the material to itself and then overlap with the previous wrap approximately 50% of the width of that particular material as wrapping progresses (Figure 1.10). This ensures sufficient coverage and even compression of the secondary bandage layer. For a typical half limb bandage with commonly used materials, this will result in the material ending where it started. If too little overlap occurs additional wraps may be needed, but if too much overlap is used there may not be enough material to finish the bandage. Tertiary bandage materials should not contact the skin and padding should be left exposed to ensure this does not occur (Figure 1.11).

Applying the Bandage

Many of the topics discussed in this chapter are concept driven. They must be realized, considered, and practiced before they can be fully understood. They are topics that may seem obvious and come as second nature to experienced individuals, but they actually are quite nuanced and somewhat complex to the novice

Figure 1.10 This cohesive bandage material is being applied in the most accepted, clockwise direction for the right front leg. Note that each wrap around the limb is applied so that it overlaps by approximately 50% the width of the previous wrap.

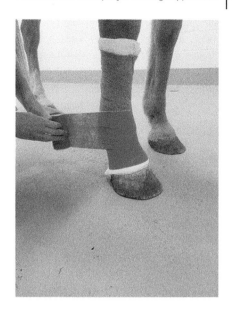

(a)

(b)

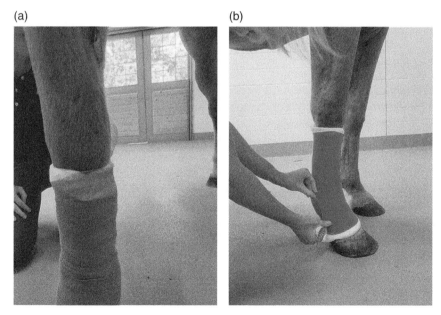

Figure 1.11 (a) The tertiary layer of bandage material (brown gauze or vet wrap) should not contact the skin. If additional tension were applied to the brown gauze and the bandage were to subsequently slip, it could cause unprotected constriction on the limb. (b) When the tertiary bandage layer is appropriately applied, approximately 1–2 cm of padding should be visible at the top and bottom of the bandage.

bandager. No matter how well one understands these topics, they are most certainly of no good if one is unable to apply them to the patient. Taking the time to consider the patient, the location, the personnel involved, and what needs to be done to prepare can make the difference between an efficient, smooth application and a chaotic, stressful situation.

Preparation for Bandage Application

When preparing for a bandage application all of the necessary materials should be gathered and laid out in an orderly fashion, with back-ups readily available, in a location within reach of where the patient will be. Inevitably, a telfa pad will be dropped or a roll gauze completely unraveled at a crucial time and a timely replacement needed. The bandage application should take place in as quiet a location as possible with ample space, free of wind, fans, dust, debris, or obstacles. The horse handler's skill should be considered in relation to the patient's temperament, as it is the handler who is keeping the bandager safe and the horse as still as possible. The need for additional assistants to hand over materials or restrain the horse should also be considered. On occasion, sedation may be necessary to help restrain the horse, protect a tenuous wound repair, or maintain the safety of everyone involved.

Safety with the Patient

When applying the bandage the horse handler and bandager should be on the same side of the horse, with the handler facing the horse and the bandager. This allows the handler to observe what is happening and to move the horse away should a dangerous situation develop. The bandager should approach the horse's shoulder from the side, make contact, and move calmly to the limb to be bandaged. The bandager should squat down, facing caudally, with both knees off the ground. This allows the bandager the best vantage point for seeing the horse and reacting to any movements, kicks, or stomps that may occur.

The assistant and any additional individuals present should remain quiet and attentive to the situation. They should be aware of what materials are being applied and in what order so they may hand them to the bandager in a timely manner. The materials should be passed over so that the bandager can grasp them and apply them to the leg without fumbling or changing their orientation. Any materials or instruments not in use should be either held by the assistant or put on an elevated surface such as a cart or table. They should not be placed on the floor surrounding the activity. Not only does this present a tripping hazard, it also provides a potential avenue of contamination that could lead to infection of a surgical site or wound (Figure 1.12).

(a)

(b)

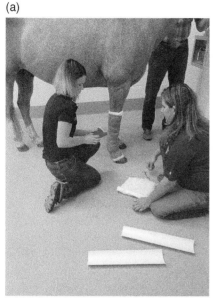 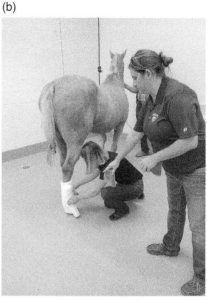

Figure 1.12 (a) Note the multiple unsafe conditions in this image. The handler is on the wrong side of the horse and backed into a corner. He cannot see what is happening, does not have room to escape, and has no safe direction to move the horse should it act out. Both the bandager and the assistant have a knee on the ground. The assistant is in front of the horse and could be struck if the horse were to act out. She also is not prepared to assist the bandager with supplies needed for subsequent steps. The bandager is facing the wrong direction and could be stepped on, run over, or kicked if the horse were to swing its back end toward her. Multiple items of bandage supplies as well as a pair of scissors are on the ground. This not only creates a tripping hazard, but also presents a risk of contamination. (b) Note the improved safety conditions compared to (a). All individuals are on the same side with room to escape. The handler and assistant are attentive to the bandager and in positions where they could move quickly. There is room to the left of the horse if it becomes nervous and needs to escape. The assistant has the needed materials in hand and ready to hand to the bandager. Note how she is holding the brown gauze with a tail so that the bandager can immediately start wrapping. The bandager is in a safe location where she can react if the horse moves.

Sweat Bandages

If a horse presents with edema in its limb and the clinician wishes to "draw out" this fluid, a sweat bandage may be applied (Figure 1.13). There are many different "sweats" that may be used. Each one seems to be unique to a certain region or discipline and can be steeped in dogma or folklore. They may be commercially available or may be concocted by the owner at home or at the veterinary clinic.

(a)

(b)

(c)

(d)

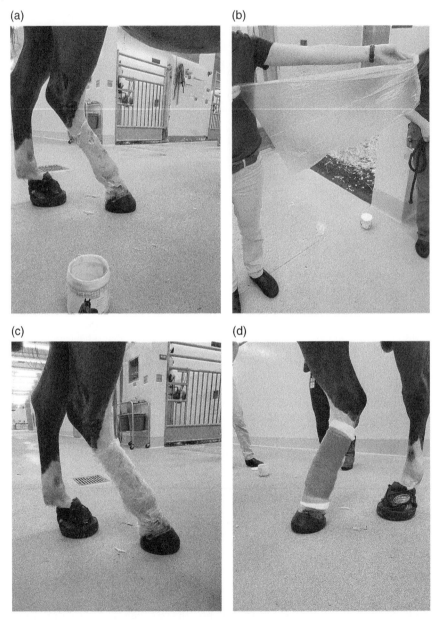

Figure 1.13 Sweat bandage application. (a) The sweat or poultice has been smeared on the edematous portion of the limb. (b) A rectal palpation sleeve has been cut open and the hand portion removed to facilitate wrapping on the leg. (c) The plastic sleeve has been wrapped on the limb over the sweat. (d) A routine half limb bandage is then placed over the plastic. This bandage is now ready for the application of cohesive and elastic bandage material.

Some are referred to as a poultice rather than a sweat or ointment. In general, they can be divided into materials considered to be either anti-inflammatory, anti-septic, hypertonic, or all of these. The examples given here are common to the authors' practice area. None seems to be more effective than any other and the choice ultimately comes down to clinician preference.

Soaking a roll of woven gauze in isopropyl alcohol is known as an alcohol sweat. The authors have often seen this applied to a horse following an extensive nerve-blocking session for lameness, where the clinician in charge hopes to avoid the development of edema and mild cellulitis.

Poultices, sometimes called muds, are commonly clay or bentonite based, mixed with various botanical or homeopathic ingredients. Many horsemen/women apply these to their horses following exercise sessions or when inflammation is expected to develop.

Another common sweat material comes in the form of various ointments or salves applied to the limb. A common commercially available product is Epsom salt based with a very thick, tenacious ointment that is green in color and has a spearmint scent. This is the authors' personal favorite, primarily because of the pleasant smell. Another common ointment-based concoction is to mix various medications, often certain amounts of a steroid, Epsom salt, and/or dimethyl sul-foxide (DMSO), in nitrofurazone ointment and apply this to the leg.

Regardless of your preferred sweat, gloves should be worn to prevent absorption into the bandager. Any open wounds should be protected with a telfa and the sweat applied liberally to the edematous areas of the leg, away from the wound. Then the leg should be covered in some form of plastic film, such as kitchen plastic wrap or a rectal sleeve slit lengthwise. A typical bandage should then be applied over the top.

Sweat bandages are typically left in place at least overnight and are usually changed within 24 hours. Sweats may be reapplied if the edema has not resolved and the clinician deems it necessary.

Special Considerations for Bandage Application

Once the bandage is applied, it is important that it be kept clean and dry. The horse should be in a stall or pen with adequate bedding and of an appropriate size to prevent it from moving excessively. The exact environment will vary with what is available to each owner and the temperament of the horse. Some horses do well in a fully enclosed 12 ft × 12 ft (3.5 m × 3.5 m) stall away from other horses. Other horses will not tolerate this and must be kept in a slightly bigger pen, outside, or with a buddy. Some owners will not have access to a stall or small pen and will need to improvise. It is important for the clinician to consider each owner's and horse's situation and to remain flexible in their recommendations to facilitate the best possible outcome.

Regardless of the environment, the bandage should be monitored at least twice daily for moisture, excessive soiling, damage, or bandage slipping. Bandages may become soaked through from an excessively exudative wound or from an overly wet environment (such as an impatient horse pawing its bucket). Many horses develop a tendency to chew or rub their bandages as their healing progresses and tissue sensations change. If a bandage becomes damaged or slips due to this, then infection or dehiscence of a surgical repair may develop. If any of these situations occur with a bandage, it should be replaced immediately with an appropriate clean, dry bandage.

Routine bandage changes should be planned for and depend on the reason for bandage application. Some bandages need to be changed daily, whereas others can remain in place for 4 to 5 days without being replaced. It is up to each individual clinician to determine bandage change frequency and make those recommendations. More frequent bandage changes allow the clinician to monitor for problems, avoid tissue macerations, and quickly address exuberant granulation tissue development, among other things. However, bandage material is costly both in money and in time/effort and it is not beneficial to change a bandage too frequently.

Typically, bloody or excessively exudative wounds are changed on a daily basis until the secondary padding layer is not being soaked through. Closed surgical incisions or laceration repairs are often changed the day following surgery and then every 2–3 days thereafter for a minimum of 14 days and sutures are removed. Incisions that dehisce or wounds managed by second intention wound healing are changed based on the amount of exudate. Often this is more frequent early in the course of healing (every 1–2 days), but can be extended as healing progress out to every 2–3, 3–4, or even 5 days depending on the nature of the wound.

An important consideration for any bandage, but particularly for horses requiring extended-duration bandaging, is how to prevent bandage sores from developing. This is primarily done by placing a consistent bandage with an even amount of tension. Even with perfect bandage placement prominences such as the accessory carpal bone and the calcaneus/calcaneal tendon are prone to developing pressure sores. These areas are managed by cutting a small slit over the prominence (accessory carpal bone), by figure-eighting bandage material around the prominence (calcaneus), or by varying the amount of tension applied over that structure. Specific techniques and recommendations will be discussed in subsequent chapters dealing with each body region.

An additional consideration for horses needing prolonged bandage application is the development of bandage-dependent edema once the wound is healed and bandaging is no longer required (Figure 1.14). This often happens in horses that have been bandaged for many weeks, but can occur with just a few days of bandaging. If the edema is mild it may be treated with benign neglect and will resolve

(a)　　　　　　　　　　　　　　　(b)

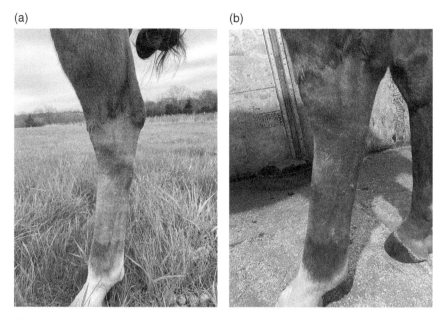

Figure 1.14   Bandage-dependent swelling. (a) A patient 14 days post surgery with the bandage having just been removed. Notice the profile of the leg and the detail of the tendons and bony prominences visible in the metatarsus. (b) The same patient 24 hours later, exhibiting mild bandage-dependent swelling. Notice the "fuller" appearance to the plantar aspect of the limb and the lack of detail of the tendons and bony prominences. This patient was addressed by 2 days of 12 hours bandage on and 12 hours bandage off, with no further bandages after that.

within a day or two. If the edema becomes pronounced or the owner is concerned, the horse may be managed with intermittent bandaging, taking a 12 hours on/12 hours off strategy for several days. This is often sufficient to resolve the issue. If edema persists, redevelops, or is concurrent with pain, the horse should be re-examined for the development of a complication or problem.

Removing a Bandage

Bandage removal may seem self-explanatory, but there are several considerations that may help expedite the process. One may simply unwrap the material from the leg and successfully remove the bandage. However, this may prove more tedious than expected given the adhesive nature of some bandage materials and the prodigious length of material used. Of course, if any of the material is to be reused, such as a polo wrap, this is the only option.

(a) (b)

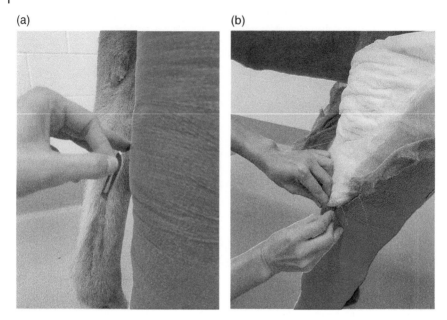

Figure 1.15 Bandage removal with a scalpel blade. (a) How to safely hold a scalpel blade to avoid cutting yourself and the horse. Notice how only a few millimeters of blade is exposed and the cutting hand is being stabilized by resting the remaining fingers of that hand on the bandage. (b) It is important to cut carefully through each layer without cutting subsequent layers underneath, especially if those layers are intended for reuse.

The next most obvious step may be to cut the tertiary layers lengthwise down the leg with bandage scissors. This also often proves more tedious than expected due to the fact that bandage scissors by design have an enlargement on one end, intended to protect the patient from impalement by the scissors. This enlargement is very effective at becoming caught within the layers of bandage material. This, coupled with the fact that bandage scissors are among the most abused instruments and subsequently become dull, can lead to a difficult process.

The most efficient way to remove a bandage is to use a disposable scalpel blade to cut the material. It is important that the bandager hold the blade in a manner to prevent a deep cut should the patient be inadvertently cut by the bandager (see Figure 1.15). Each layer of bandage material is carefully cut and removed.

Bandage Management and Complications

Bandages should be monitored closely (at least twice per day) and kept clean and dry at all times. They should be changed at regular intervals as dictated by the nature of the wound or incision in order to monitor for the development of

Figure 1.16 This patient was bandaged with only cohesive bandage material directly on the skin to cover a minor abrasion. On presentation to the veterinary clinic swelling had begun to accumulate proximal to the bandage. Fortunately, only minor discomfort was present. The swelling resolved with appropriate bandaging and systemic anti-inflammatory medication without developing any more serious complications.

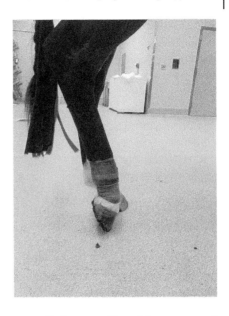

complications. Bandages that slip or become soiled or wet (due either to wound exudate or to external sources) should be changed as soon as possible. Horses should remain in a confined space to limit limb motion, which promotes bandage slippage and the development of bandage-related sores.

Bandages that are not monitored closely or are applied incorrectly have a higher chance of developing bandage-related complications. The primary cause of many complications is the pressure exerted by the bandage material on the limb. When uneven or excessive tension is used during bandage application or when slippage occurs and pressure is applied at unintended areas, the underlying tissues can become injured (Figure 1.16). At a minimum this pressure promotes accumulation of edema, and tissue swelling fosters local inflammation and interferes with tissue healing.

When uneven pressure is applied over the flexor tendons, a stress point is created at the junction between high and low pressure. This can lead to tendon injury, commonly known as a "bandage bow" because the swollen injured tendon takes on a curved appearance and bows palmarly/plantarly. Mild bandage bows are simply accumulations of edema with mild tenderness, whereas severe bandage bows result from actual damage to the tendon fibers themselves or disruption of the blood supply to the area. The mild injuries are self-limiting and can be managed with local cold therapy, anti-inflammatory medication, and application of an appropriate bandage for several days until resolved. The severe injuries can cause substantial lameness and should be assessed via ultrasound to determine the best approach to treatment. This may include an extended rest and rehabilitation period to allow the injured tendon to heal.

An additional consequence of uneven pressure or excessive pressure with insufficient padding is local disruption of the blood supply and subsequent skin necrosis. Often this presents as moderate pain and swelling in the area, but progresses over several days to sloughing of the skin over the potentially large affected area (Figure 1.17). Once this occurs the skin needs to be managed via second intention wound healing and this can have a substantial negative impact on the patient.

A particular area where skin pressure sores can occur is over bony prominences such as the accessory carpal bone, the point of the hock, or at the margin of a bandage where high motion occurs such as the calcanean tendon. Typically these complications do not develop during short periods of bandaging (7–10 days), but prolonged periods of bandaging can lead to the development of these sores (Figure 1.18). In cases where a long period of bandaging is known from the outset, relief cuts can be made through the tertiary bandage layers over the bony prominences to relieve the pressure. Even then, sores may not be prevented.

When sores do occur, the owner should be informed and warned that white hairs may develop in the area as a result. Often, the cases that develop pressure sores need continued bandaging due to the nature of their primary injury, and the only recourse for the bandage sores is to provide appropriate wound treatments.

(a)

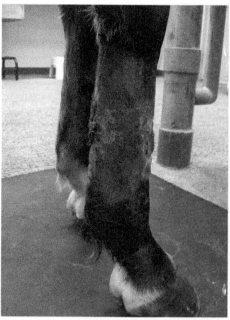

Figure 1.17 This patient presented for sloughing of the skin on the dorsal and palmar aspects of its right front metacarpus due to bandage-induced pressure necrosis. Ten days prior it had developed pain and swelling in the area after having a bandage placed by one of the barn employees. The patient subsequently ruptured the common digital extensor tendon as a result of the injury, but went on to heal with second intention wound management. (a) Lateral view of the bandage pressure necrosis wound on presentation.

(b)   (c)

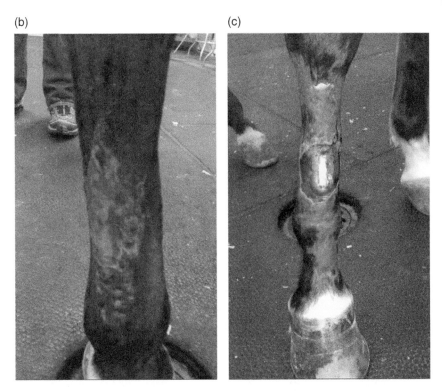

Figure 1.17 (Continued) (b) Palmar view of the wound over the flexor tendons. (c) Dorsal view of the wound over the extensor tendon and third metacarpal bone.

In some cases some of the bandage may be cut away to relieve pressure over the sore or a creative wrapping pattern used to avoid pressure in the area. Often these sores persist and may worsen until bandaging is discontinued.

Finally, a particular complication related to bandaging foals is the development of flexor tendon laxity and a dropped (hyperextended) fetlock as a result of the bandage. The flexor tendons provide support to the limb through the action of their muscle bellies. When a bandage is applied to a foal limb, the material itself provides support to the limb and the flexor muscles do not need to work as hard. Subsequently these become weakened to the point that they are unable to adequately support the fetlock after bandage removal. If this occurs, the foal should be exercise restricted until the muscles regain strength and the addition of a heel extension shoe considered. The heel extension functions by providing a longer lever arm at the sole of the foot for the tendons to pull on. This longer lever reduces the force needed to fully support the fetlock.

(a) (b)

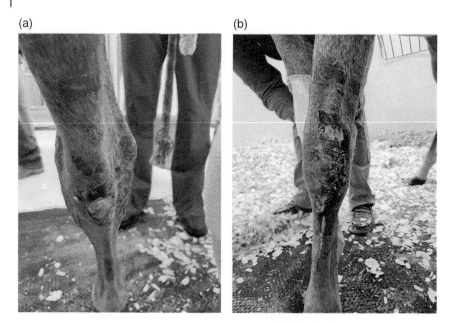

Figure 1.18 (a) Skin pressure necrosis over the accessory carpal bone in a six-month=old foal being managed for a severe carpal laceration over several weeks. (b) Skin pressure necrosis over the medial epicondyle of the radius at the proximal aspect of the sutured laceration. Notice the hardened, leathery appearance of the skin surrounding the sore. This indicates that skin has been injured by the pressure. It subsequently went on to slough.

Suggested Reading

Theoret, C. and Schumacher, J. (ed.) (2017). *Equine Wound Management*, 3e. Ames, IA: Wiley.

Chapter 5: Topical Wound Treatments and Wound Care Products by Stine Jacobsen

Chapter 6: Update on Wound Dressings: Indications and Best Use by Stine Jacobsen

Chapter 7: Bandaging and Casting Techniques for Wound Management by Yvonne A. Elce

2

Distal Limb Bandages

The equine distal limb is the most commonly bandaged area of the horse. There are multiple types of bandages that may be applied, depending on the reason for bandaging. This chapter covers multiple tips, tricks, and nuances that will improve the appearance and quality of the bandage. The supplies required are listed in Tables 2.1 and 2.2.

Hoof Bandages

A hoof bandage, sometimes called a boxing glove bandage because it encompasses the entire foot, is useful for covering not only the hoof structures but also the areas around the coronary band and distal pastern (Figure 2.1). The primary use of this bandage is for managing hoof abscesses, where a soaking bandage can be created by placing a 5 L fluid bag over the foot and covering it with the bandage material (Figure 2.2). This bandage is also particularly helpful for very distal wounds or incisions where a routine half limb bandage may allow contamination to work its way proximally from the ground. An inexpensive and readily available alternative to using a combine cotton roll is to place a diaper around the foot instead. It is important to prepare a duct tape pad to be placed over the bottom of the bandage (Figure 2.3). This will prevent the horse from wearing through the bandage material as it moves in its stall.

Application of the hoof bandage is described in Figure 2.4.

Equine Bandaging, Splinting, and Casting Techniques, First Edition. J Dylan Lutter, Haileigh Avellar, and Jen Panzer.
Companion website: www.wiley.com/go/lutter/1e

Table 2.1 Supply list for foot bandage.

Material needed	Number needed
Cotton combine roll – cut square to fit foot	1 square
6 in. brown gauze	1 roll
4 in. cohesive bandage	1 roll
Duct tape	1 roll, construct a patch to fit the foot
Materials needed for a foot soaking bandage	
Loose roll cotton	Small amount; roughly 5–10 cm length
Epsom salts	½–1 cup
Empty 5 L fluid bag	1 bag
10% betadine solution	10–20 ml

Table 2.2 Supply list for half limb bandage.

Material needed	Number needed
Cotton combine roll	1 roll, pre-packaged or self-cut to approx. 50 cm length
6 in. brown gauze	1 roll
4 in. cohesive bandage	1 roll
Elastic adhesive tape	1 roll
Materials needed only if wound or incision is present	
4 in. sterile woven gauze	1 roll
Telfa pad	1 pad sized to cover wound or incision

(a) (b)

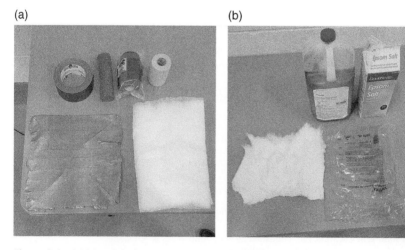

Figure 2.1 (a) Materials for a hoof bandage. (b) Materials for a foot soaking bandage.

Figure 2.2 This soaking bandage is useful for soaking horses with hoof abscesses or puncture wounds. The goal is to soften the sole to facilitate abscess rupture or to make it easier to pare away the sole with a hoof knife. These bandages are more convenient (and less messy) for soaking than standing the horse in a bucket. They can be left in place for 12 hours or more before they need to be changed. Oftentimes one overnight soak is sufficient, but a soak bandage can be replaced if necessary. (a) Cut off the bottom of the 5 L fluid bag that contains the fluid line ports. It is important to remove this portion because the port will have been punctured for patient administration and would leak if left in place. Then place the cotton roll in the bag. A small amount will go a long way. Using too much cotton will make for an unusually bulky bandage. (b) Add the Epsom salts and 10% betadine solution to the bag. Only a small amount of either is necessary. While only a splash of betadine is commonly added without measuring, the best practice would be to make a 0.1–0.2% dilute betadine solution by adding 10–20 ml of betadine to 980–990 ml of water. *Be certain that it is solution and not scrub.* The scrub contains detergents that are detrimental to wound healing and will also create foam that will overflow the fluid bag as the horse moves.

(a)

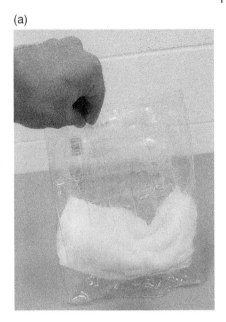

(b)

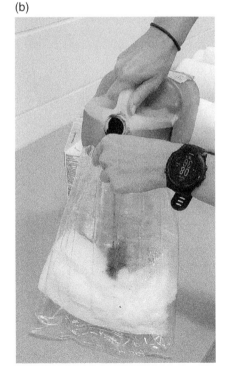

(c)

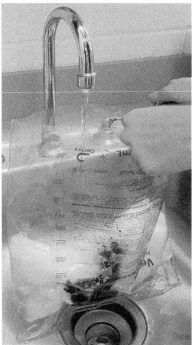

Figure 2.2 (Continued) (c) Add only enough tap water (or your newly mixed dilute betadine solution) to the bag to fully moisten the cotton. A few hundred milliliters should be sufficient. Adding too much water will cause the bag to overflow when the horse stands on the bandage. (d) Carefully place the horse's foot in the bag and replace it in a weight-bearing stance. Use duct tape or elastic tape to secure the bag to the horse's leg. If this is not done, the horse may easily step out of the bag and spill the contents as you are preparing for the rest of the foot bandage.

(d)

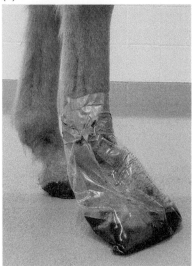

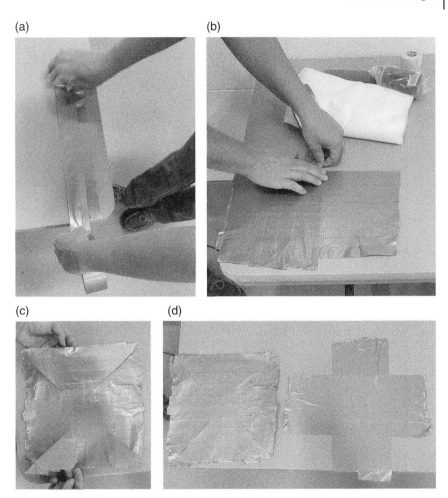

Figure 2.3 The duct tape pad is made by overlapping eight to nine strips in roughly a square. This will be sufficiently large for most patients except for the largest warmbloods and draft horses. (a) It is helpful to make the pad on a counter with a sharp edge to facilitate cleanly tearing the tape as shown here. (b) A second layer of eight to nine overlaid tape strips is placed at 90° to the first. Additional layers may be added if necessary. The authors have had to use pads up to five layers thick for large draft horses housed in concrete-floored stalls. (c) Relief cuts in an X pattern are made to all the edges to fold up around the bandaged hoof. It is important to leave an uncut center area that is slightly larger than the bottom of the foot being bandaged. (d) An alternative style of duct tape pad is to make a plus sign with enough strips so that the two overlapped layers are the size of the foot. This style uses less tape and does not need to be cut prior to application of the foot.

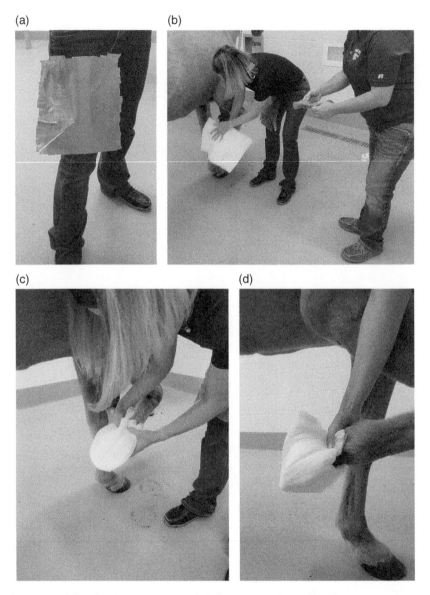

Figure 2.4 A foot bandage may be applied directly over the soaking foot, separately over a dressing applied to the hoof, or over a wound in the distal pastern region where it is desirable to completely seal off the foot from the environment. (a) Once made and lifted off the table, it is very easy for the duct tape pad to stick to itself. If there is not an assistant available, a handy way to keep it safe and close by is to stick it to the bandager's leg while the rest of the bandage is being applied. (b) To begin the foot bandage, the horse's foot is lifted and held by the bandager's hand that is closest to the horse. The bandager's contralateral hand drapes the cotton combine square over the foot, taking care to center it. Notice in this image that the assistant stands at the ready to hand over the next piece of bandage material or to step in and lend a hand holding the leg if needed. (c) The cotton square is then folded around the hoof, fully enclosing it. (d) The bandager holds the corners of the cotton square in one hand around the pastern and reaches for the brown gauze roll. All of the subsequent steps should be done as swiftly as possible without setting the foot down.

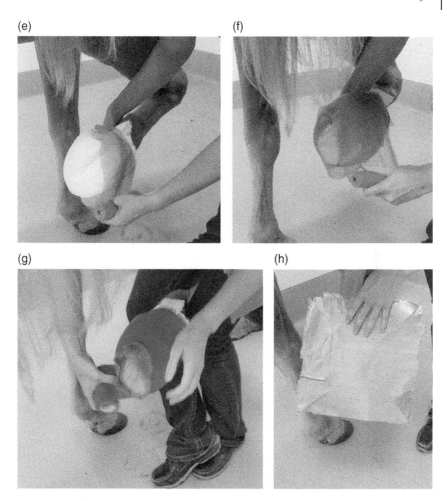

Figure 2.4 (Continued) (e) The bandager holds the tail of the brown gauze with the same thumb that is holding the leg and uses the other hand to wrap two to three times circumferentially around the hoof and pastern. The step is necessary to compress the cotton and secure the bandage to the leg. (f) Once secured to the leg, the brown gauze is wrapped, crisscrossed, and figure-eighted to fully compress the cotton and cover the bottom of the foot as many times as possible. Because the hoof capsule is so rigid, a large amount of tension is not vital for this layer. (g) Once the brown gauze roll is applied, the same process is repeated for the cohesive bandage layer, taking two to three wraps circumferentially then crisscrossing to fully compress the cotton and cover the bottom of the foot. Enough tension should be applied to remove the crinkles from the material and ensure that it sticks to itself. (h) Next, the duct tape pad is placed, centered on the bottom of the foot. At this point the foot could be placed on the ground, but oftentimes the pad will inadvertently either fall off or become stuck to itself when this is being done. If possible, it is best to keep holding the foot.

(i) (j)

(k) (l)

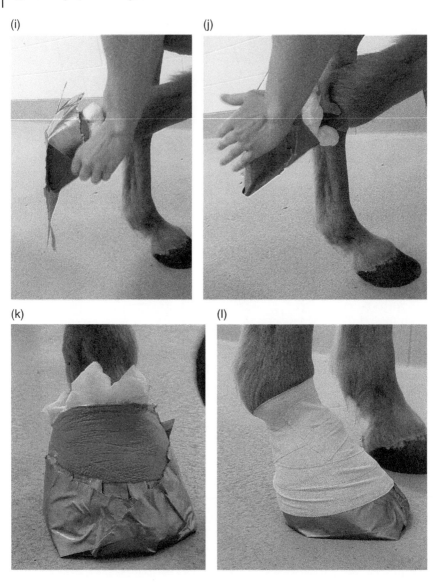

Figure 2.4 (Continued) (i) The tabs of the tape pad are folded up around the foot to secure the pad in place. (j) If the square style of pad with the X cut is used, the "wings" of each tab can be wrapped around each other and will fully enclose the bandage in duct tape. (k) The foot may then be placed on the ground and additional duct tape added if needed to fully secure the tape pad. This often is needed if the tabs become folded onto themselves or if the plus sign style pad is used. (l) The bandage is finished by sealing the top to the skin with elastic tape. Any loose ends or gaps in the duct tape may also be secured at this time.

Half Limb Bandages

The half limb bandage is the most commonly used bandage for horses, primarily because the distal limb in horses commonly sustains wounds, injuries, or trauma (Figure 2.5).

Positioning the Cotton Combine Padding

Cotton combine padding can be purchased in a wide variety of widths. It can be purchased in bulk 10 yard lengths and cut at the clinic, or purchased already cut, rolled, and packaged for individual use. Commonly clinics only purchase one or two widths that will best fit the size of horses most commonly seen in the area. Since each cotton will not fit every horse perfectly, clinicians must consider how best to place the cotton on the limb to provide a reasonable bandage that fits the horse well.

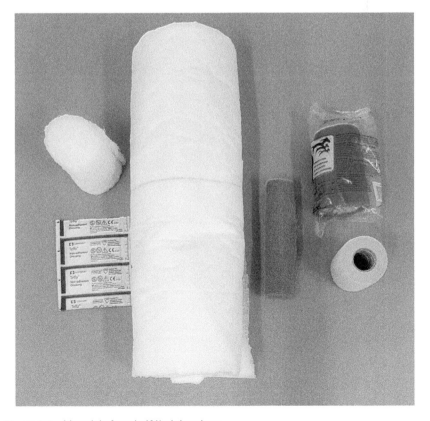

Figure 2.5   Materials for a half limb bandage.

The bandager needs to consider where the top and bottom margins of the cotton will lie in relation to the horse's anatomy and any wounds or incisions that are present. Figure 2.6 illustrates common positions of the cotton roll.

Applying the Half Limb Bandage

Application of the primary layers (telfa pad and woven gauze, if needed) will not be covered in this section. The reader is referred to Figure 1.1 for an illustration of how they are applied. Following placement of the primary layer, the secondary (padding) layer is applied while taking into consideration its positioning on the limb. Finally, the materials for the tertiary layer are applied to secure the bandage. Figure 2.7 illustrates this process and provides additional tips/techniques. Figure 2.8 shows a finished half limb bandage.

(a)

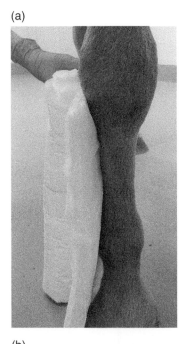

(b)

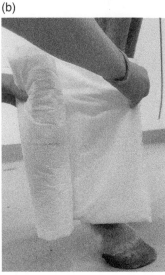

Figure 2.6 Positioning considerations for the cotton combine rolls in a half limb bandage. (a) The first thing to consider is where the top margin of the cotton lies in relation to the carpus or tarsus of the horse. In general it is best if the cotton ends before contacting a high-motion portion of the carpus/tarsus, usually within the proximal metacarpal/metatarsal region. (b) Next, the bottom margin should be considered. For most wounds within the metacarpal/metatarsal region, the bottom margin of the cotton can be placed roughly in the mid-pastern region, but it can be shifted further distally to accommodate appropriate placement of the top margin.

(c)

(d)

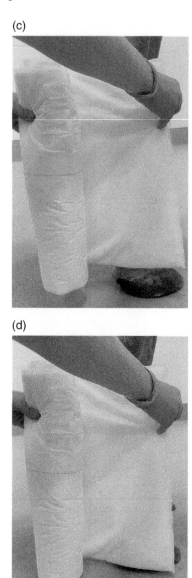

Figure 2.6 (Continued) (c) If a wound or incision is within the fetlock region it may be best to move the cotton a bit further distally to end at the level of the coronary band. Though this is a seemingly small difference from (b), it improves the stability of the bandage and helps prevent dirt/debris from migrating proximally under the bandage. (d) Finally, if a wound is present in the pastern region or even near the coronary band, the cotton can be shifted further distally to rest on the ground. This ensures maximal coverage of the most distal aspect of the limb and is often more easily applied than a foot bandage. With this positioning, special attention should be paid to the top margin of the cotton. If it is too low (i.e. ending in the mid-cannon bone region) a wider cotton roll should be used.

Figure 2.7 Application of a half limb bandage to a front limb. This illustrates cotton placement at the level of the coronary band. The same technique can be applied to the rear limb. (a) The half limb bandage begins with the bandager positioning the cotton roll in relation to the carpus and distal limb structures (refer to Figure 2.6 for more information). The end of the roll is secured with one hand and the cotton wrapped neatly around the limb without tension being applied, but in a relatively snug fashion so that the margins align well and there are no areas that are excessively bulky or bulging. (b) The finished secondary layer is held with one hand while the bandager retrieves the next bandage material. Note the even alignment of the top and bottom margins as well as the relatively uniform appearance of the bandage at this point.

(a)

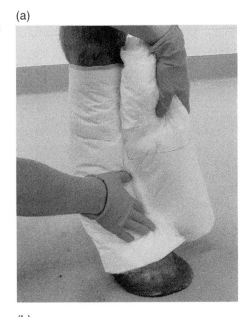

(b)

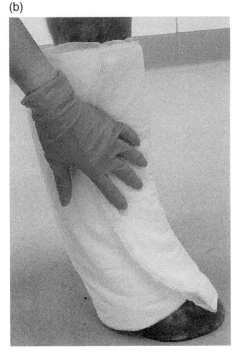

(c)

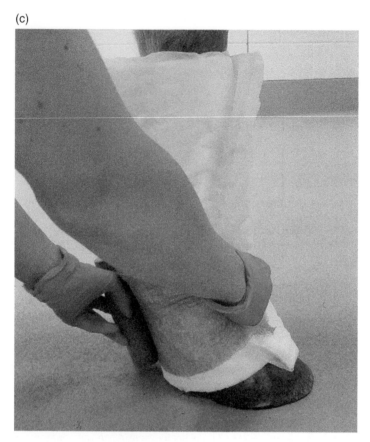

Figure 2.7 (Continued) (c) The tertiary layer is started by holding the tail of the brown gauze. In this example, the bandager has chosen to begin the bandage at the bottom but, as noted in Chapter 1, it does not make a substantial difference where to start this layer and it is up to each individual to decide. Some bandagers will tuck this tail beneath the final wrap of the cotton roll to help hold it more securely. One full wrap around the leg is taken before tension is applied to the brown gauze so that it will bind on itself and hold the tension.

(d)   (e)

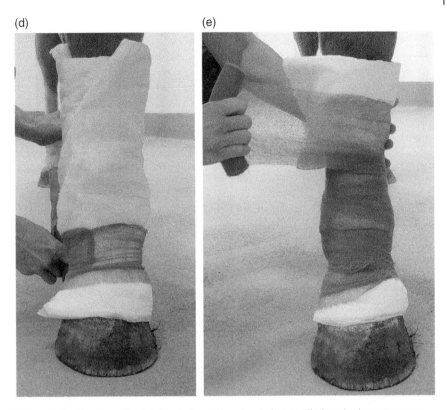

Figure 2.7 (Continued) (d) A front view of tension being applied to the brown gauze after the initial wrap around the leg. Notice how the cotton is compressing. Also notice how the distal margin of gauze has slid proximally, exposing an additional amount of cotton padding. This commonly occurs because of the contour of the leg at this location and is an acceptable amount if bandaging for a wound in the fetlock region or more proximally. However, if the bandage is being applied for a wound in the pastern or even coronary band region, these may not have sufficient compression without taking additional wraps slightly more distally with the brown gauze. Sufficient and even compression is important because it reduces the risk of bandage-induced tissue trauma. Additionally, the lack of compression may allow for proximal migration of dirt/debris or even sliding of the bandage to expose a very distal wound. (e) Consistent, even tension is applied to the brown gauze while wrapping the limb with approximately 50% overlap of the width of the gauze roll. The bandager should strive to achieve approximately 80% of the desired cotton compression with tension from the brown gauze. More compression is often not achievable because the gauze is easily torn. Notice how the gauze roll is bending and conforming to the bandager's hand as she is pulling on it. This may lead to the tendency for the gauze to bunch up as it unrolls and is applied to the limb. This bunching places uneven pressure and reduces the coverage of the material as it is being applied. To combat this, the bandager may grasp the bottom edge of the gauze and pull distally to spread out this tension and apply the gauze more evenly. This is being demonstrated in (g).

(f)   (g)

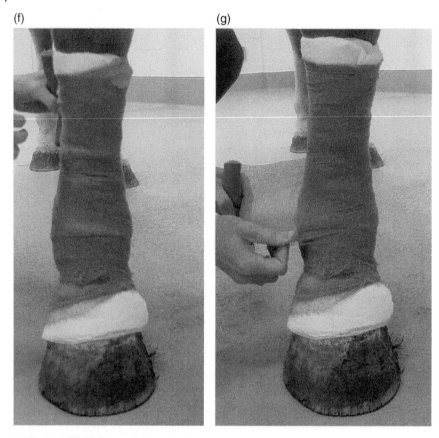

Figure 2.7 (Continued) (f) Once the gauze has reached the top, leaving a small amount of cotton showing, the bandager continues to wrap distally again with the same 50% width overlap. Notice how the distal margin of the brown gauze has slipped proximally on the medial aspect despite the attempts to prevent this. Deliberate application of the cohesive bandage over this area will help address the uneven compression. (g) Continued application of the brown gauze. Here the bandager demonstrates how to grasp the gauze and spread the pressure from the tension for more wide and uniform compression of the cotton. Notice the more compressed and uniform contour of the bandage at this stage compared to earlier photos in the sequence. This is a good indication of appropriate bandage application thus far.

Figure 2.7 (Continued) (h) The appearance of the bandage after finishing the brown gauze layer. Notice the even contour of the limb and the small amount of cotton showing at the top and bottom of the bandage. If a brief pause is needed at this stage, the brown gauze will often cling to itself momentarily or a corner at the end of the roll can be tucked into the bandage to hold it. The bandager should not delay application of the cohesive bandage unnecessarily, as any movement from the horse will cause the bandage to unravel. (i) Here the cohesive bandage layer is being applied with 50% width overlap. Just prior to the picture, the tail was applied using one wrap around the limb with just enough tension for the material to stick to itself. Then additional tension was applied until the crinkles disappeared and the material took on a smoother appearance. This represents roughly 60–70% of the tension the material can sustain and will achieve the remaining compression of the cotton padding to result in a sturdy bandage. Notice how the uncompressed cotton from earlier in the sequence has been sufficiently compressed by this layer.

(h)

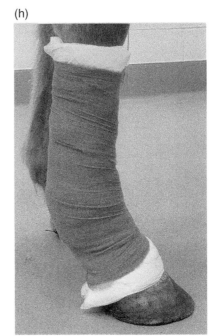

(i)

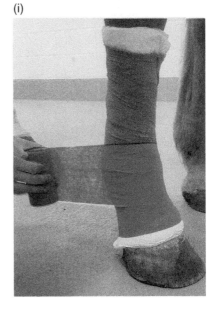

(j)

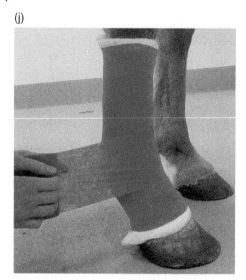

Figure 2.7 (Continued) (j) Continued application of the cohesive bandage material. The bandager reached the top of the cotton, leaving approximately a finger's width showing, and continued to wrap back down the leg. (k) The tertiary layer has been completed and elastic tape is being applied to seal the ends of the bandage. Not shown is that roughly half the width of the tape was initially applied to the bandage and the other half applied to the skin/hoof. One and a half to two wraps are typically sufficient to seal the bandage. If the bandager desires a better distal seal, the limb may be picked up and tape wrapped below the heel bulbs, as this is a common area for dirt/debris to gain access.

(k)

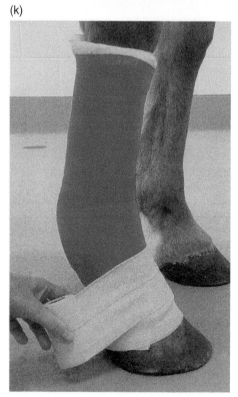

(l)   (m)

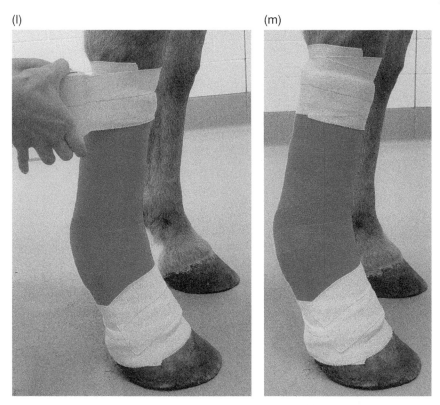

Figure 2.7 (Continued) (l) The top of the bandage is being sealed in a similar fashion with half the tape applied to the bandage and half applied to the skin. Take note here that little to no tension should be applied to the tape to prevent unprotected constriction of the bandage material. (m) The finished half limb bandage. Notice the uniform, compressed appearance of the bandage that follows the contours of the limb. If one were to flick the bandage at this point it would sound somewhat hollow, like flicking a ripe watermelon. This is an indication that a stout bandage has been applied with adequate tension on the bandage material.

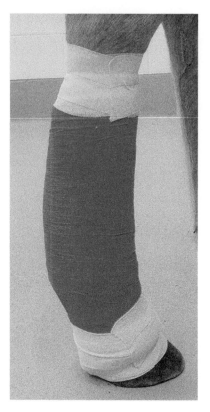

Figure 2.8 The appearance of a finished half limb bandage placed on a hind limb. Notice that the top margin of the bandage ends before the high-motion region of the tarsus.

3

Full Limb Bandages

Front Limb

The full limb bandage is used for horses when they sustain injuries to their carpus, antebrachium, and tarsus. These bandages are commonly referred to as "stack" bandages due to the stacking position of cotton rolls. The materials required are illustrated in Figure 3.1 and listed in Table 3.1.

Application of the primary layers (telfa pad and woven gauze, if needed) will not be covered in this section. The reader is referred to Figure 1.1 for an illustration of how they are applied. Following placement of the primary layer, the secondary (padding) layer is applied while taking into consideration its positioning on the limb. Finally, the materials for the tertiary layer are applied to secure the bandage. Figure 3.2 illustrates this process and provides additional tips/techniques.

Rear Limb

Like for the front limb, application of the primary layers (telfa pad and woven gauze, if needed) to the rear limb will not be covered in this section. The reader is referred to Figure 1.1 for an illustration of how they are applied. Following placement of the primary layer, the secondary (padding) layer is applied while taking into consideration its positioning on the limb. Finally, the materials for the tertiary layer are applied to secure the bandage. Figure 3.3 illustrates this process and provides additional tips/techniques.

Equine Bandaging, Splinting, and Casting Techniques, First Edition. J Dylan Lutter, Haileigh Avellar, and Jen Panzer.
© 2024 John Wiley & Sons, Inc. Published 2024 by John Wiley & Sons, Inc.
Companion website: www.wiley.com/go/lutter/1e

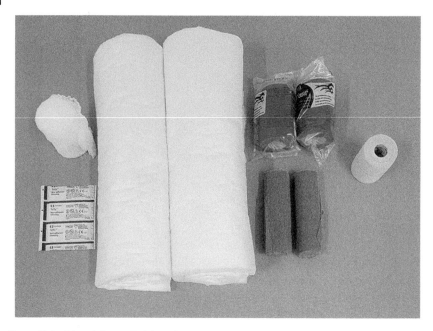

Figure 3.1 Materials needed for a full limb bandage are similar to those for a half limb, except that the amounts of secondary and tertiary layer materials are doubled.

Table 3.1 Supply list for half limb bandage.

Material needed	Number needed
Cotton combine roll	2–2.5 rolls, pre-packaged or self-cut to approx. 50 cm length
6 in. brown gauze	2 rolls
4 in. cohesive bandage	2 rolls
Elastic adhesive tape	1 roll
Materials needed only if wound or incision is present	
4 in. sterile woven gauze	1 roll
Telfa pad	1 pad sized to cover wound or incision

Figure 3.2 Application of the full limb bandage to the front limb. (a) The full limb bandage begins with positioning the cotton combine roll from the coronary band to the distal carpus. This cotton roll should be applied snuggly. Brown gauze is applied in the same direction as the cotton combine roll and even tension is applied to the limb. A small amount of cotton combine is left exposed at the top and bottom of the bandage. Refer to Figure 2.7a–h for further instructions. (b) A second cotton combine roll is stacked on top of the distal limb bandage with 2–4 in. (5–10 cm) overlap. Notice in this image that the second cotton roll is being applied over the distal limb bandage without the cohesive bandage layer in place. Once the proximal brown gauze is applied, two rolls of cohesive bandage will be applied over the entire bandage to bind the layers together, making a fully enclosed bandage. An alternative approach would be to first apply the cohesive bandage layer to the distal bandage before proceeding to the proximal bandage. This alternative is illustrated in Figure 3.3.

(a)

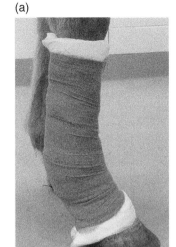

(b)

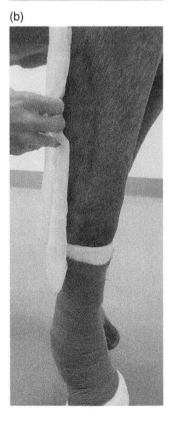

(c)

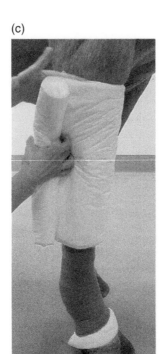

(d)

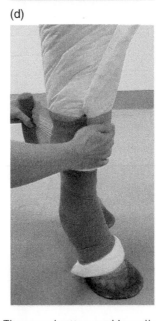

Figure 3.2 (Continued) (c) The second cotton combine roll should be placed snugly around the upper limb and in the same direction as the distal limb cotton and brown gauze. Note the even alignment of the upper and lower margins and even appearance of the bandage. The upper portion of the secondary layer is held in place while retrieving the tertiary layer materials. (d) The tertiary brown gauze layer begins at the distal portion of the upper combine roll with one to two wraps securing the cotton in place.

Figure 3.2 (Continued) (e) Following the initial wrap the brown gauze should move slightly distally to cover all the overlapping portions of the cotton combine roll. Tension to the brown gauze after the initial wrap around the leg should be applied evenly and compression of the cotton should be noticeable. (f) Consistent, even tension is applied to the brown gauze while wrapping the limb with approximately 50% overlap of the width of the gauze roll. The bandager should strive to achieve approximately 80% of the desired cotton compression with tension from the brown gauze. More compression is often not achievable because the gauze is easily torn. If insufficient compression is placed on this layer it can lead to bandage slippage, increased movement of the limb, and migration of debris into the bandage. Bunching of the bandage can occur with uneven tension and pressure during placement of the tertiary layer. This is combatted by grasping the bottom edge of the brown gauze and gently pulling distally to spread the tension evenly. This is demonstrated in Figure 2.7g.

(e)

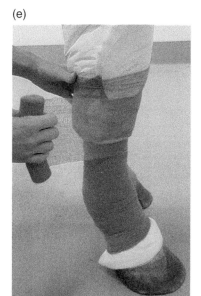

(f)

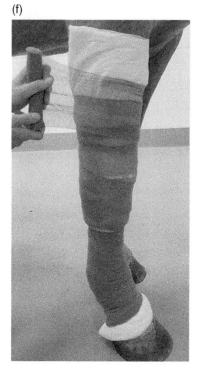

(g)

(i)

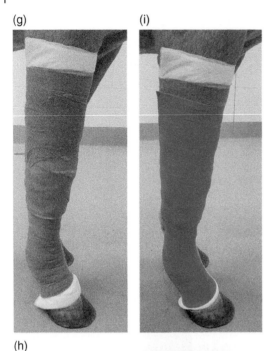

(h)

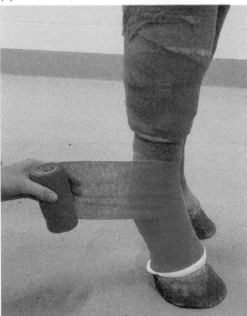

Figure 3.2 (Continued) (g) The appearance of the bandage after finishing the brown gauze layer. Notice the even contour of the limb and the small amount of cotton showing at the top and bottom of the bandage. If a brief pause is needed at this stage, the brown gauze will often cling to itself momentarily or a corner at the end of the roll can be tucked into the bandage to hold it. The bandager should not delay application of the cohesive bandage unnecessarily, as any movement from the horse will cause the bandage to unravel. (h) The cohesive bandage layer is being applied with 50% width overlap. Just prior to the picture, the tail was applied using one wrap around the limb with just enough tension for the material to stick to itself. Then additional tension was applied until the crinkles disappeared and the material took on a smoother appearance. This represents roughly 60–70% of the tension the material can sustain and will achieve the remaining compression of the cotton padding to result in a sturdy bandage. (i) The cohesive bandage material is continued up the limb with even tension and 50% overlap of the material. In full limb bandages two rolls of cohesive material are typically needed to cover the entire tertiary layer.

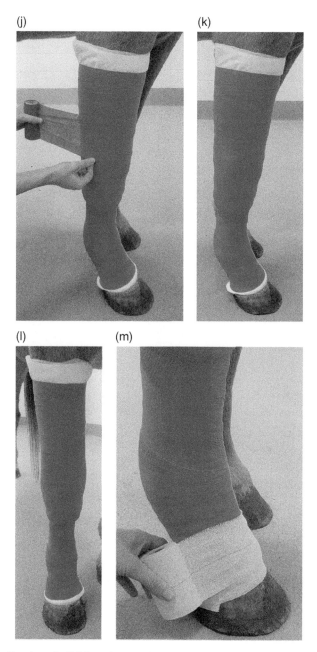

Figure 3.2 (Continued) (j) When the top of the bandage is reached, approximately 1 in. (2.5 cm) of cotton combine roll is continued to be wrapped down the leg. (k) The completed bandage prior to elastic tape placement. (l) View from the dorsal aspect of the bandage prior to elastic tape placement. (m) The tertiary layer has been completed and elastic tape is being applied to seal the ends of the bandage. Not shown is that roughly half the width of the tape was initially applied to the bandage and the other half applied to the skin/hoof. One and a half to two wraps are typically sufficient to seal the bandage. If the bandager desires a better distal seal, the limb may be picked up and tape wrapped below the heel bulbs, as this is a common area for dirt/debris to gain access.

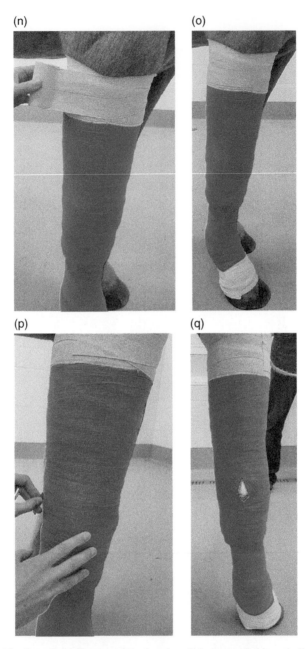

Figure 3.2 (Continued) (n) The top of the bandage is being sealed in a similar fashion with half the tape applied to the bandage and half applied to the skin. Take note here that little to no tension should be applied to the tape to prevent unprotected constriction of the bandage material. A full two to three wraps may be needed at the top of full limb bandages to help keep them in place. (o) The finished full limb bandage. Notice the uniform, compressed appearance of the bandage that follows the contours of the limb. (p) A properly applied bandage places compression across the entire forelimb. Excessive compression across the accessory carpal bone can lead to trauma and skin necrosis on this aspect of the limb. Due to this it is recommended to incise through the cohesive and tertiary layers, releasing the compression directly over this portion of the palmar aspect of the carpus. (q) The finished full limb bandage of the forelimb with release of compressive layers over the accessory carpal bone.

(a)   (b)

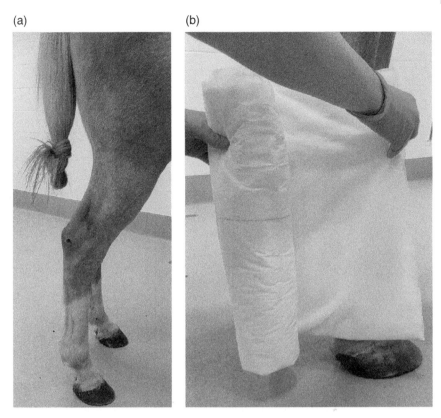

Figure 3.3 Application of the full limb bandage to the hind limb. (a) Positioning the patient is very important when placing all bandages. For application of a full limb hind limb bandage, the horse should be standing squarely underneath itself, as demonstrated in this picture. The patient's tail is secured in a knot; additional material such as tape or cohesive bandage may be used to keep the tail out of the way during the bandaging process. (b) Primary, secondary, and tertiary layers should be placed in a routine fashion. Refer to Figure 2.8.

(c) (d)

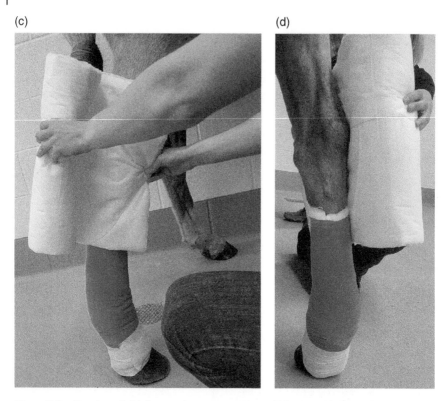

Figure 3.3 (Continued) (c) A second cotton combine roll is placed overlapping the distal bandage by approximately 2–4 in. (5–10 cm). The combine roll should be placed in the same direction as the distal layer. Notice in this image that the proximal combine roll is being applied over the distal bandage that has the cohesive layer in place. This approach is an alternative to that illustrated in Figure 3.2. The main advantage of this approach is that the proximal and distal bandages are maintained separately. If desired, the proximal bandage could be changed to care for a wound while the distal bandage was maintained, in order to save the money, time, and effort required for the distal bandage. With this approach, the distal bandage is typically changed every other bandage change. (d) An additional image of the 2–4 in. (5–10 cm) overlap of the proximal combine roll over the distal bandage. Notice that the elastic tape has not been placed in the proximal metatarsus.

Figure 3.3 (Continued) (e) The tertiary brown gauze layer begins at the distal portion of the upper combine roll with one to two wraps securing the cotton in place. (f) Consistent, even tension is applied to the brown gauze while wrapping the limb with approximately 50% overlap of the width of the gauze roll. The bandager should strive to achieve approximately 80% of the desired cotton compression with tension from the brown gauze. More compression is often not achievable because the gauze is easily torn. If insufficient compression is placed on this layer it can lead to bandage slippage, increased movement of the limb, and migration of debris into the bandage. Bunching of the bandage can occur with uneven tension and pressure during placement of the tertiary layer. This is combatted by grasping the bottom edge of the brown gauze and gently pulling distally to spread the tension evenly. This is demonstrated in Figure 2.7g. Some bandagers will use a figure-eight pattern over the point of the hock to decrease tension on this area. This technique can be seen in (j) and Figure 5.2c–f with the placement of the cohesive layer and tarsal bandages. If the figure-eight technique is not used as in this image, it is important to use slightly decreased tension while placing the brown gauze layers over the point of the hock. The authors strive to achieve three successive wraps of brown gauze over the point of the calcaneus to achieve a strong bandage in that area. Other techniques of reducing tension in this area that are not shown here include placing cotton pads to the medial and lateral aspects of the gastrocnemius tendon, then completing the bandage as described next.

(e)

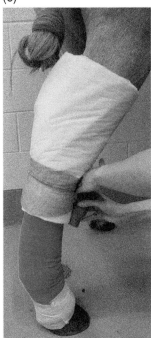

(f)

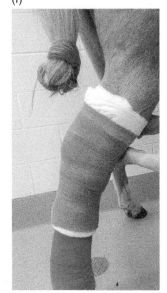

(g)

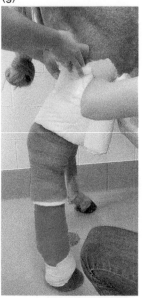

(h)

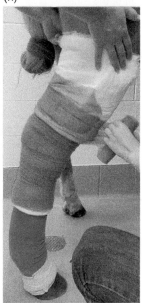

Figure 3.3 (Continued) (g) Additional full or partial cotton combine rolls may be needed to fully cover the limb, depending on the size of the horse and the injury it has sustained. The third combine roll is placed in a similar manner as previously described. It should be wrapped in the same direction as the previous layers and fit snugly with no excessive folds in the material. An assistant is often needed to help keep this layer in place. In cases where two combine rolls are sufficient, skip to (i). (h) Tertiary brown gauze is placed as previously described, leaving approximately 1 in. (2.5 cm) of cotton exposed at the proximal aspect. An assistant may be needed to keep bandage layers in place.

(i)

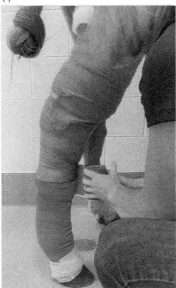

(j)

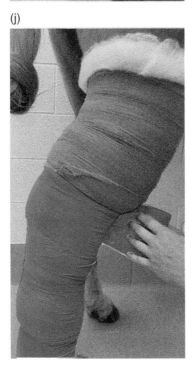

Figure 3.3 (Continued) (i) The cohesive bandage layer is applied with 50% width overlap starting at the distal aspect of the bandage. Tension is applied until the crinkles disappear and the material takes on a smoother appearance. (j) A cohesive bandage layer placed in a figure-eight technique over the point of the hock and not pulling the material to its fullest extent. This is to decrease the pressure of the bandage at the point of the hock. If too much pressure is applied it can lead to skin trauma and necrosis, as well as cause the horse to be uncomfortable in the bandage. Multiple rolls of cohesive material are usually needed to complete a full limb bandage. Approximately 1 in. (2.5 cm) of cotton should remain at the top of the bandage.

(k) (l)

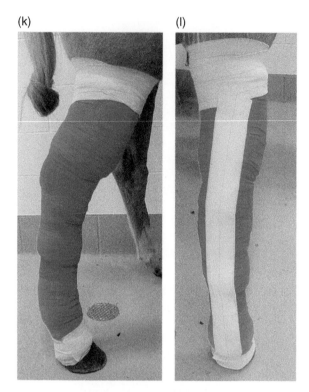

Figure 3.3 (Continued) (k) Elastic tape is placed at the distal and proximal aspects of the bandage as described in Figure 3.2m,n. (l) Full limb bandages greatly restrict the range of motion of the hind limb, but due to the reciprocal apparatus of the horse, many horses do not tolerate the restricted movement initially and will hyperflex their hock and kick out, causing disruption of the caudal aspect of the bandage. This may occur immediately after bandage placement, during recovery from anesthesia, or getting up and down in a stall. It is advised that the bandager and horse handler are aware of this risk and are able to quickly move to a safe location and not get kicked while the horse adjusts to the bandage. An additional technique used by many bandagers includes placing a full-length strip of elastic tape from the proximal to distal aspects of the bandage to reinforce its most vulnerable area.

4

Carpal Bandages

Carpal bandages are typically reserved for wounds or incisions located in the carpal region, but may also be used for covering the proximal metacarpus or distal radius. These bandages have a propensity to loosen and slip because of the tapered profile of the equine forearm and the lack of supporting bandage material in the distal limb. Often a full limb bandage is placed in instances where a carpal bandage could be used because of the reduced risk of the bandage slipping.

This bandage is particularly sensitive to inadequate tension being placed on the bandage material. This will result in premature slippage of the bandage and require more frequent bandage changes. Nevertheless, in situations where one wishes to reduce the amount of bandage material used or where the distal limb is desired to be uncovered, a carpal bandage can be useful.

The materials required for a carpal bandage are illustrated in Figure 4.1 and listed in Table 4.1. Figure 4.2 outlines the method of application.

Equine Bandaging, Splinting, and Casting Techniques, First Edition. J Dylan Lutter, Haileigh Avellar, and Jen Panzer.
© 2024 John Wiley & Sons, Inc. Published 2024 by John Wiley & Sons, Inc.
Companion website: www.wiley.com/go/lutter/1e

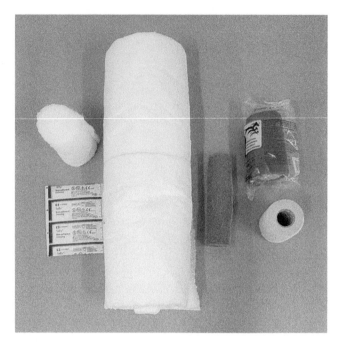

Figure 4.1   Materials for a carpal bandage.

Table 4.1   Supplies needed for a carpal bandage.

Material needed	Number needed
Cotton combine roll	1 roll, pre-packaged or self-cut to approx. 50 cm length
6 in. brown gauze	1 roll
4 in. cohesive bandage	1 roll
Elastic adhesive tape	1 roll
Materials needed only if wound or incision is present	
4 in. sterile woven gauze	1 roll
Telfa pad	1 pad sized to cover wound or incision

Figure 4.2 Application of an equine carpal bandage. (a) After the primary contact layer is applied (not shown), the secondary cotton padding is applied in the standard fashion, centered over the carpus. As with other bandages, this layer does not need to be applied tightly. It should be rolled onto the leg so that the top and bottom margins are neatly aligned, without any areas of excessive bulk. (b) Once the secondary layer is finished the tertiary layer is begun similarly to the distal limb bandage. A single wrap with minimal tension is used to bind the brown gauze on itself. Then enough tension is applied to substantially compress the cotton. Starting the brown gauze layer at the bottom of the bandage will help to uniformly compress the cotton and act to anchor the bandage in place as the compression is moved proximally. If, for some reason, the bandager prefers to begin the brown gauze over the carpus, minimal difficulties should arise. If this approach is taken, it is strongly suggested to wrap the brown gauze distally first. Difficulties will arise if the brown gauze layer is started at the proximal aspect of the bandage, because the angled contour of the horse's forearm will promote bandage slippage as compression is applied to the first few wraps.

(a)

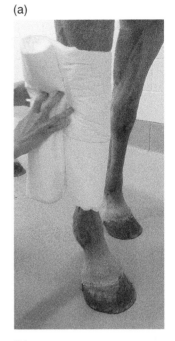

(b)

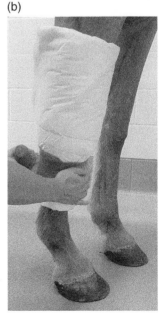

(c)

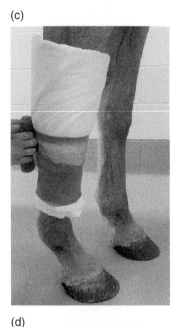

(d)

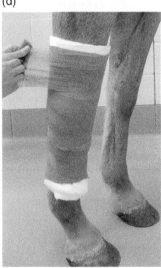

Figure 4.2 (Continued) (c) The brown gauze is continued to be wrapped in a proximal direction with the standard overlap of 50% of the width of the gauze roll. Even tension should be maintained with each wrap of the gauze. As with the half and full limb bandages, enough pressure should be applied to achieve roughly 80% of the achievable compression. (d) The brown gauze continues to be wrapped until the top of the cotton is reached, stopping with roughly a finger's width of cotton still showing. The brown gauze is then wrapped distally until the roll is fully applied.

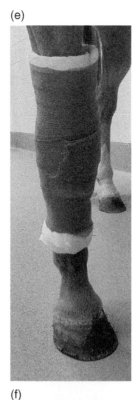

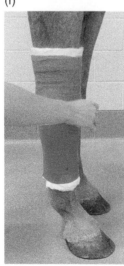

Figure 4.2 (Continued) (e) The finished appearance of the brown gauze layer. Note the compressed appearance of the cotton, which nicely conforms to the leg. (f) The cohesive bandage layer is begun in a similar fashion to the brown gauze, being sure to leave a small amount of cotton showing. Enough tension is applied to remove the crinkles from the material and give it a smooth appearance. This layer is wrapped proximally with the same 50% width overlap.

(g)

(h)

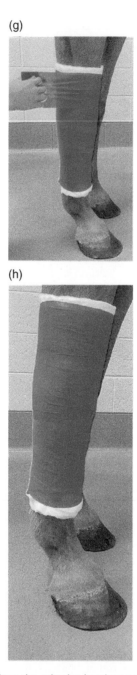

Figure 4.2 (Continued) (g) Once the cohesive bandage reaches the top of the cotton, it is continued by wrapping distally, being sure to leave a small amount of cotton visible. (h) A side view of the bandage with the finished tertiary layer.

(i) (j)

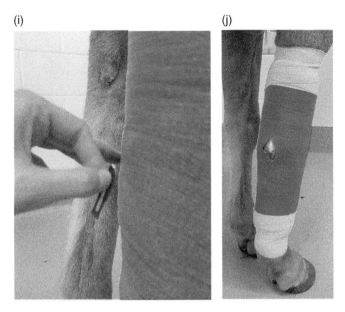

Figure 4.2 (Continued) (i) Once the tertiary layer is completed, the bandager may optionally elect to make a relief cut over the accessory carpal bone. If the cut is not made there is a chance of pressure sore development in cases requiring prolonged bandaging. This cut should continue through the cohesive and brown gauze layers to expose the cotton but not disrupt it. The cut should be roughly 2–4 cm in length. Notice how the bandager is holding the scalpel blade and bracing her fingers on the bandage to stabilize during the cut. This will help prevent accidentally cutting too deeply. (j) A rear view of the finished carpal bandage. In this image the elastic tape has already been applied. Adding one to two additional wraps of the elastic tape, compared to a half limb bandage, on the top and bottom of the bandage will give additional anchoring to the bandage and may reduce slipping. Notice the size and depth of the relief cut made over the accessory carpal bone.

5

Tarsal Bandages

Tarsal bandages are typically used for wounds or incisions located in the tarsal and calcaneal regions. These bandages have a propensity to loosen, slip, and be disrupted or tear at the caudal aspect of the bandage due to hyperflexion of the tarsus following bandage application. Often a full limb bandage is placed in instances where a tarsal bandage could be used because of the reduced risk of the bandage slipping.

This bandage is particularly sensitive to both inadequate tension being placed on the bandage material and excessive tension over the tuber calcaneus or point of the hock. This will result in premature slippage of the bandage and require more frequent bandage changes. In situations where one wishes to reduce the amount of bandage material used or where the distal limb is desired to be uncovered, a tarsal bandage can be useful.

The materials required for a tarsal bandage are illustrated in Figure 5.1 and listed in Table 5.1. Figure 5.2 details the method of application.

Equine Bandaging, Splinting, and Casting Techniques, First Edition. J Dylan Lutter, Haileigh Avellar, and Jen Panzer.
© 2024 John Wiley & Sons, Inc. Published 2024 by John Wiley & Sons, Inc.
Companion website: www.wiley.com/go/lutter/1e

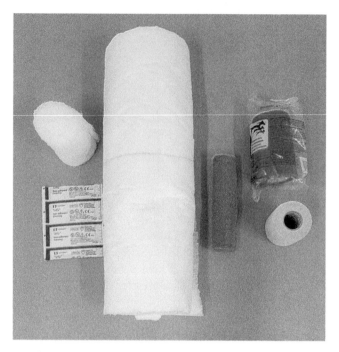

Figure 5.1 Materials for placement of a tarsal bandage.

Table 5.1 Supplies list for tarsal bandage.

Material needed	Number needed
Cotton combine roll	1 roll, pre-packaged or self-cut to approx. 50 cm length
6 in. brown gauze	1 roll
4 in. cohesive bandage	1 roll
Elastic adhesive tape	1 roll
Materials needed only if wound or incision is present	
4 in. sterile woven gauze	1 roll
Telfa pad	1 pad sized to cover wound or incision

(a)   (b)   (c)

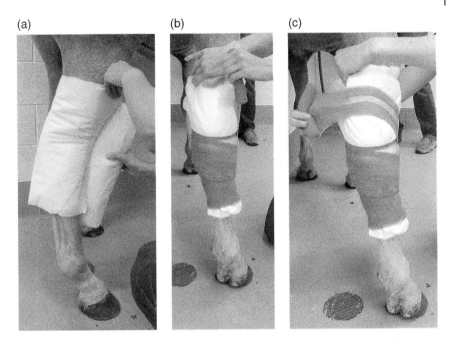

Figure 5.2 Application of an equine tarsal bandage. (a) A primary contact layer is applied (not shown) before the secondary cotton padding is applied in a standard fashion, centered over the tarsus. As with other bandages, this layer does not need to be applied tightly. It should be rolled onto the leg so that the top and bottom margins are neatly aligned, without any areas of excessive bulk. (b) Once the secondary layer is finished the tertiary layer is begun, similarly to the distal limb bandage, with 50% overlap. A single wrap with minimal tension is used to bind the brown gauze on itself, then enough tension is applied to substantially compress the cotton. Starting the brown gauze layer at the bottom of the bandage will help to uniformly compress the cotton and act to anchor the bandage in place as the compression is moved proximally. (c) Many bandagers prefer to use a figure-eight technique over the point of the hock. This decreases the tension on the tuber calcaneus, which is a common location for bandage sores to develop. Excessive tension over the calcanean tendon should also be avoided. The brown gauze should be crossed at the dorsal aspect of the tarsus with several layers placed distal and proximal to the point of the hock.

(d)   (e)   (f)

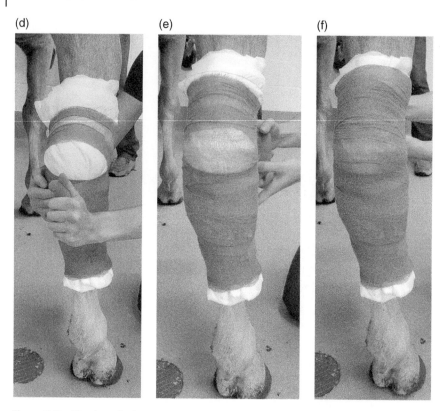

Figure 5.2 (Continued) (d) Ensuring placement of the brown gauze by using the figure-eight technique with approximately 50% overlap on the proximal and distal portions of the bandage. (e) One to two layers of brown gauze can be placed over the point of the hock with minimal to no tension, which acts as another layer in the event of tearing of the bandage in this location. Some bandagers prefer to leave the point of the hock free from brown gauze. (f) The finished application of brown gauze leaving approximately 1 in. (2.5 cm) of cotton combine roll free at the proximal and distal aspects of the bandage.

(g)

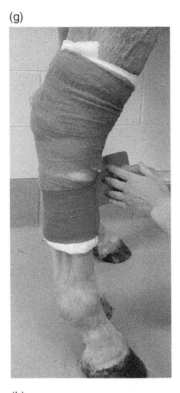

(h)

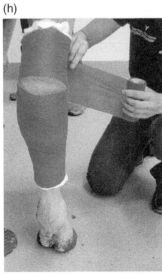

Figure 5.2 (Continued) (g) Application of cohesive material starting at the distal aspect of the bandage. There should be 50% overlap of the material moving proximally. (h) A figure-eight technique should be used with the cohesive layer, as described with the brown gauze in (c–e). Minimal tension should be placed over the point of the hock.

(i)

(j)

(k)

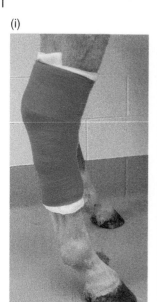
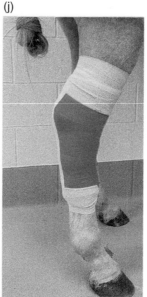
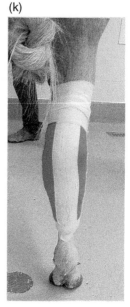

Figure 5.2 (Continued) (i) The finished cohesive layer of the tarsal bandage. Approximately 1 in. (2.5 cm) of cotton should be visible at the top and bottom of the bandage. (j) Placement of elastic tape should be at the top and bottom of the bandage to help prevent dirt and debris from entering and decrease the risk of slippage. This technique is described further in Figures 3.2m,n and 3.3k. (k) An additional full-length elastic tape strip is often placed at the plantar aspect of the bandage to decrease the risk of bandage tearing. This is further described in Figure 3.3l. Some horses react negatively to the restricted movement of the tarsus immediately after application of the bandage. The bandager and horse handler should be aware of the situation and able to quickly move to a safe location to avoid getting kicked.

6

Head and Neck Bandages

The equine head and neck are commonly wounded areas. Not every wound or incision in these areas needs to be bandaged and many heal well without a covering. There are times, however, when a bandage is necessary to maintain the cleanliness of a wound or where a bandage may improve the cosmetic outcome of a wound. Being able to think creatively and construct a bandage for unconventional areas is a good skill to develop. This chapter illustrates three of the more commonly used bandages in the authors' experience.

The materials required for a head or neck bandage are illustrated in Figure 6.1 and listed in Table 6.1.

Ear Bandage

Wounds to the ear are relatively uncommon in horses, but when they do occur the injury often affects the shape and contour of the ear. Applying a bandage to this damaged tissue will help maintain the ear's shape and improve both the functional and the cosmetic outcome for the horse. The series of images in Figure 6.2 utilizes a roll of gauze to help with the ear's contour. The authors have also fashioned stiff plastic stents made from baseball cap bills or plastic pails and sutured these to the ear, through the ear cartilage, with reasonable success in cases where an ear deformity developed from a laceration.

Head Pressure Bandage

A head pressure bandage (Figure 6.3) is often useful following enucleation or to bandage a wound that enters the frontal sinus. A creative wrapping pattern around the head is necessary to secure the bandage in place while also ensuring

Equine Bandaging, Splinting, and Casting Techniques, First Edition. J Dylan Lutter, Haileigh Avellar, and Jen Panzer.
© 2024 John Wiley & Sons, Inc. Published 2024 by John Wiley & Sons, Inc.
Companion website: www.wiley.com/go/lutter/1e

(a)

(b)

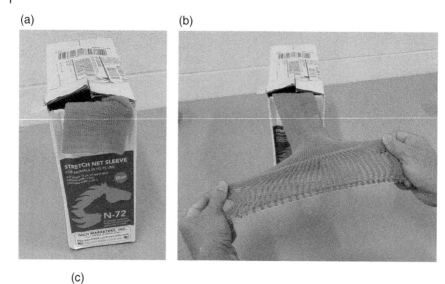

(c)

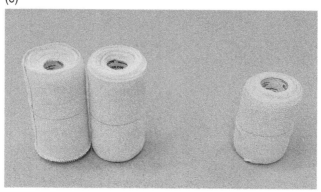

Figure 6.1 (a–c) Materials for placing a bandage on the head or neck.

Table 6.1 Supplies list for head/neck bandage.

Material needed	Number needed
Distensible netting	Length and diameter variable, depending on need
Elastic adhesive tape	1–2 rolls, depending on need
2 in. woven gauze – optional	1 roll
6 in. brown gauze – optional	1 roll
Materials needed only if wound or incision is present	
4 in. sterile woven gauze	1 roll
Telfa pad	1 pad sized to cover wound or incision

(a)

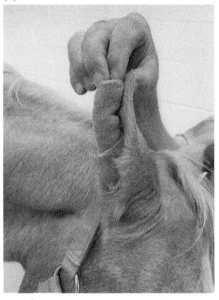

(b)

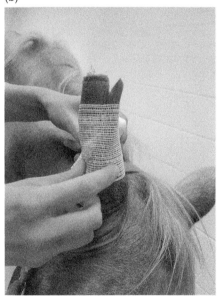

Figure 6.2 An example of an ear bandage that may be used to help maintain the contour of an injured ear or place pressure if needed to reduce edema or a hematoma. (a) Roll gauze is placed on the inner surface of the pinna to help maintain the inner contour and prevent the pinna from collapsing when wrapped. A 6 in. brown gauze is pictured here, but this may result in an excessively long and unwieldy bandage, as seen later in this sequence. A narrower width of gauze may be used if support all the way to the tip of the pinna is not needed. (b) The gauze roll is secured in place by several wraps of 2 in. woven gauze, commonly called conforming gauze. Minimal tension should be applied when wrapping. This layer also helps to protect the sensitive ear from the elastic tape to be applied in the next step.

(c)

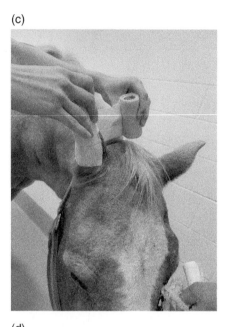

(d)

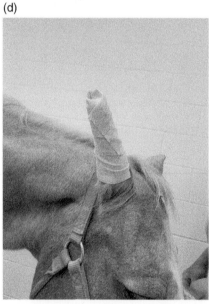

Figure 6.2 (Continued) (c) Elastic tape is wrapped around the ear to secure the gauze in place. Again, minimal tension should be applied when wrapping. (d) The appearance of the sealed ear bandage. Depending on the situation, this may be all that is needed. However, there is little holding the bandage in place and additional measures may need to be taken to secure the bandage and support the ear against the extra weight of the bandage material.

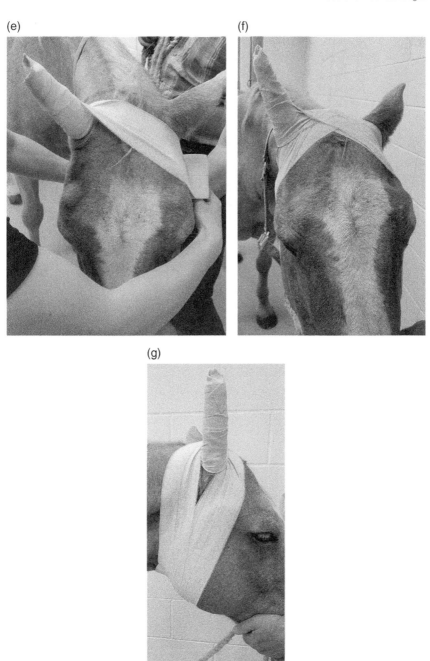

Figure 6.2 (Continued) (e) If additional security and support of the ear are desired, the elastic tape may continue to be wrapped in a figure-eight pattern around the ear, under the throat latch/jaw of the horse. (f) The finished front appearance of the ear bandage. (g) The finished side appearance of the ear bandage.

(a)

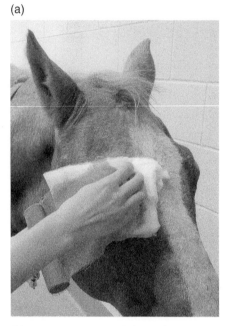

Figure 6.3 Application of a head pressure bandage. (a) A dressing is applied to any incision or surgical wound. Here 4 x 4 in. gauze squares are being used as if the patient were being bandaged following a standing enucleation. The dressing may be secured in place by roll gauze to increase patient comfort when removing the bandage. The use of the gauze does reduce bandage security, making it easier for the patient to rub the bandage off. (b) A bandage dressing held in place with roll gauze. Note the figure-eight pattern with gauze located in front of and behind the ramus of the mandible. If additional bandage security is desired, more gauze may also be rolled further caudally around the neck, caudal to the ears.

(b)

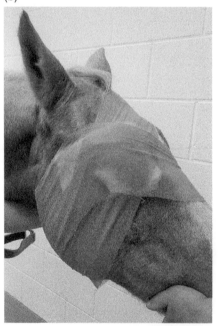

(c)

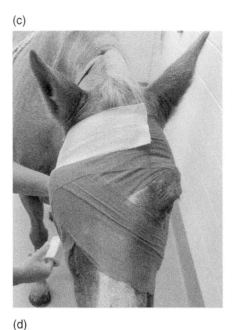

(d)

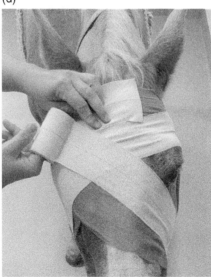

Figure 6.3 (Continued) (c) Next, elastic tape is applied to further secure the dressing and gauze in place. Notice that the patient's unaffected eye is not incorporated into the bandage and that the elastic tape is being applied half onto the hair and half onto the gauze. (d) The elastic tape is figure-eighted around the head in a similar fashion to the roll gauze, being careful not to impinge on the patient's unaffected eye.

(e) (f)

(g)

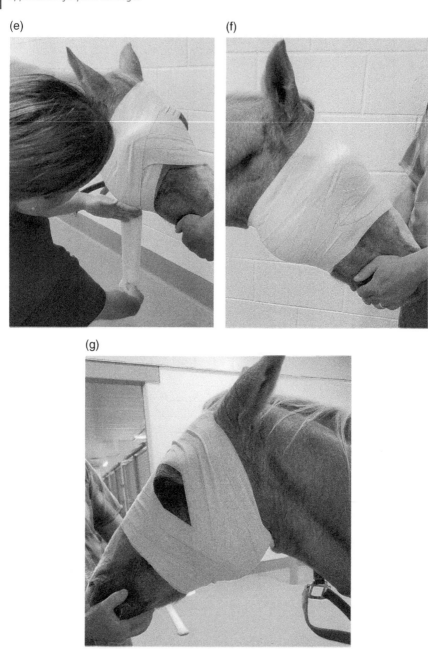

Figure 6.3 (Continued) (e) Continued wrapping with elastic tape. Here a new roll of tape is being applied with the end secured just out of view on the left side of the patient's forehead. (f) The finished side appearance of a head pressure bandage. Note that if additional bandage security were desired, the elastic tape could be wrapped caudal to the ears around the neck. (g) The finished appearance from the side of the unaffected eye, illustrating how this eye is not impinged on.

that the ears and unaffected eye are not covered. Some horses are very adept at rubbing the bandage off. Additional wraps caudal to the mandible may be needed as well as those shown in this sequence.

Head Netting Bandage

A situation may present itself where a head wound or incision is desired to be covered but where no pressure is necessary or pressure may even be detrimental to healing (Figure 6.4). A good example would be a horse with a depression fracture of the frontal bone that has been elevated back into place and a wound over this area. Additional pressure from a bandage may result in destabilizing and re-depressing the fracture fragment. In this instance, a netting bandage may be applied (Figure 6.5). An alternative material to use would be 4 or 5 in. diameter cast stockinet, which is also easily stretched and could be rolled onto the horse's head.

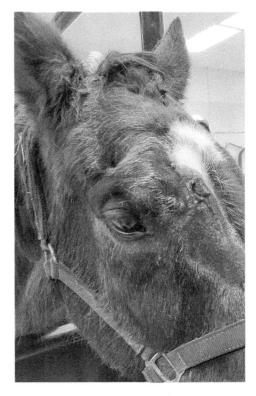

Figure 6.4 An example of a patient where a netting bandage would be useful. This horse has a semi-circular incision that was placed to facilitate a trephine hole into the frontal sinus for standing lavage.

(a) (b)

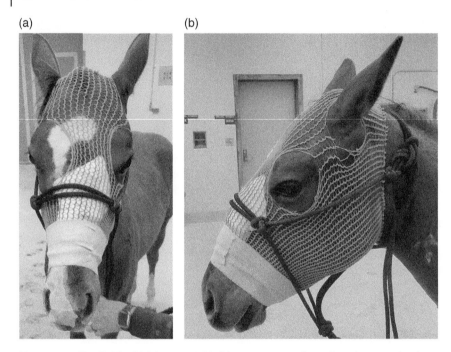

Figure 6.5 The finished (a) front and (b) side appearance of a patient that sustained a wound to the bridge of its nose that required wound dressing. This netting is easily torn or cut to create ear and eye holes. It may be secured in place using elastic tape or left free.

7

Upper Limb and Body Bandages

Wounds on the upper limb and body are common. These locations can be difficult or impossible to bandage with the techniques listed in the previous chapters. Not every wound or incision in these areas needs to be bandaged and many heal well without a covering. There are times, however, when a bandage is necessary to maintain the cleanliness of a wound, reduce tension on the wound repair, or where a bandage may improve the cosmetic outcome of a wound. This chapter illustrates the more commonly used bandages in the authors' experience.

Elastic Tape/Ether Bandage

An elastic tape/ether bandage is useful for the protection of surgical site incisions or minor wounds that are not otherwise easily bandaged and could benefit from being covered (Figure 7.1). The authors find one particularly useful following laparoscopic surgery with small incisions in the paralumbar fossa or after stifle arthroscopy. These bandages often remain in place for several days if applied immediately post-operatively when the skin is clean, well clipped and prepped, and dry. Once the horse is returned to its stall and the skin begins to become soiled by the environment, these bandages tend not to adhere as well.

Equine Bandaging, Splinting, and Casting Techniques, First Edition. J Dylan Lutter, Haileigh Avellar, and Jen Panzer.
© 2024 John Wiley & Sons, Inc. Published 2024 by John Wiley & Sons, Inc.
Companion website: www.wiley.com/go/lutter/1e

(a)

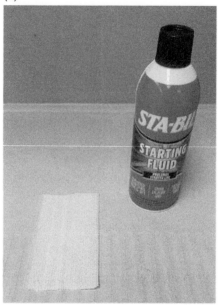

(b)

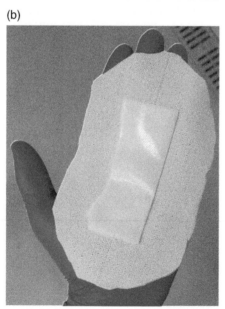

Figure 7.1 Application of a simple elastic tape/ether bandage. (a) The bandager begins by cutting a strip of elastic tape long and wide enough to cover the desired area. Bandages approximately the length of one's hand are typically the largest that can be easily applied. If available, laboratory-grade ether should be gathered for use, but if unavailable aerosol starting fluid purchased at the automotive store is as effective. This ether is to be sprayed/poured onto the adhesive tape, which begins to melt the adhesive and increases its stickiness. (b) A strip of non-adherent wound dressing is cut to fit within the confines of the tape of sufficient size to cover the intended incision. Here, a telfa pad is being used. The edges of the adhesive tape are trimmed to remove any corners, jagged edges, and the very edges of the tape that do not contain adhesive. The goal here is to help promote a smooth, continuous seal circumferentially around the bandage.

(c)

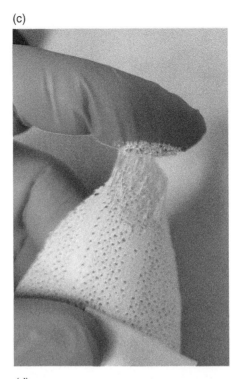

(d)

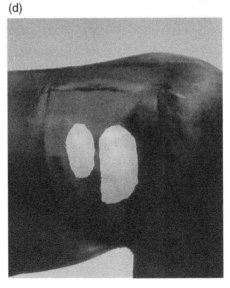

Figure 7.1 (Continued) (c) Immediately prior to application on the patient, the ether is applied to the adhesive tape. It is unavoidable that the telfa pad will become soaked with ether. This will quickly evaporate and will not negatively impact the incision it is covering. The image here illustrates how the ether is melting the adhesive and increasing its stickiness. Once the ether has been applied the bandage should be placed on the patient immediately. If the ether is allowed to dry it ruins the adhesive and a new bandage needs to be made. (d) The final appearance of the bandage, which was placed over laparoscopy portal incisions following completion of standing surgery in this patient.

Tie-Over Bandage

A tie-over bandage is another useful bandage for the proximal limb and body regions (Figure 7.2 and Table 7.1). It is best suited for securing wound dressings and applying pressure to often bulky materials to hold them in place.

(a)   (b)

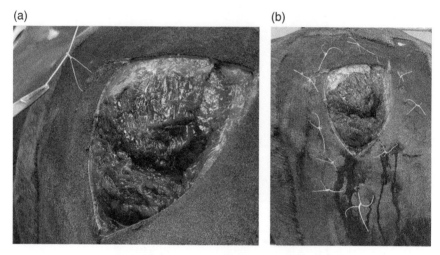

Figure 7.2 Application of a tie-over bandage on a large gluteal wound. (a) A tie-over bandage is secured to the patient by lacing umbilical tape through loops of suture that have been placed around the wound. These sutures are placed after the appropriate wound treatment has occurred and any wound closure has been performed. The skin is sterilely prepped and sites for suture placement blocked with subcutaneous injection of local anesthetic. The suture for the loops should be non-absorbable and of sufficient size so that they do not break when tension is applied. This is typically a minimum of size 1 (4.0 metric) suture or larger. The loops should be left large enough that the umbilical tape can be easily threaded through them using gloved fingers without having to pull or tug on the patient, but they should not be left so large that they will touch each other once the lacing is tightened. (b) An example of the location and spacing of suture loops prior to bandaging. Note that they are several centimeters from the wound margin so that they do not interfere with any wound care that needs to occur at a later time. The loops have roughly been placed in pairs, one on each side of the wound, and more loops than is necessary are in place. Often, after several days of bandaging the loops pull out of the skin. Having extra loops in place initially can be useful in preventing the need to re-sedate, re-block, and re-place new loops.

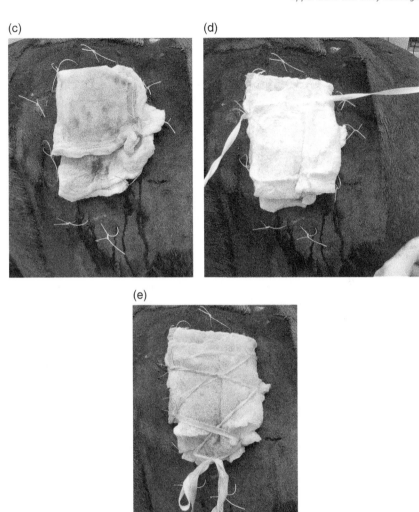

Figure 7.2 (Continued) (c) The intended wound dressing and secondary bandage layer are applied. Here saline-soaked woven gauze laparotomy sponges are being used as the primary bandage layer in the application of a wet–dry bandage that will debride any debris and devitalized tissue when it is removed the following day. (d) Umbilical tape 0.25 in. wide is threaded through the suture loops to secure the bandage material. Note that a dry gauze laparotomy sponge has been applied as the secondary bandage material layer. (e) The finished tie-over bandage. The umbilical tape has been laced in a shoelace pattern and tied in a bow at the bottom with sufficient extra tape. This pattern and placement facilitate later loosening of the umbilical tape so that the wound dressing and bandage material may be changed without fully removing the tape. The umbilical tape can easily be cut and removed if it becomes too soiled and stiff.

Table 7.1 Materials needed for placement of a tie-over bandage.

Material needed	Number
#0–#2 non-absorbable suture	1–2 packs, depending on size of wound
Local anesthetic (lidocaine, carbocaine)	1 bottle
Surgical tools (needle drivers, suture scissors)	1 each
Combine cotton roll	1
Umbilical tape	Variable length

Abdominal Wrap

A circumferential elastic tape bandage is typically applied to cover large incisions or wounds on the ventral or lateral aspects of the abdomen or even thorax (Figure 7.3 and Table 7.2). It is particularly useful in creating a tight seal over incisions from abdominal exploratory or colic surgery. While there are commercial "belly" bandages manufactured for this use, it is not feasible in many cases to have all sizes in stock. In some situations the manufacturing delay to make the bandage does not match the short duration for which a bandage may be needed. In those situations it is necessary to apply an elastic tape bandage.

(a)

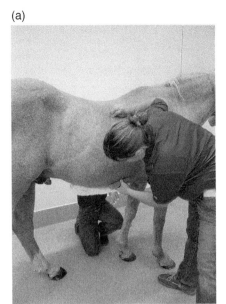

(b)

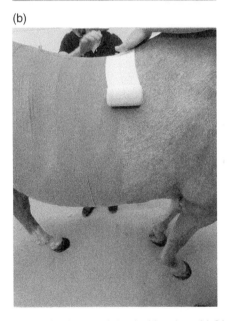

Figure 7.3 Application of an elastic tape abdominal bandage. (a) Oftentimes these bandages are applied because of abdominal fluid drainage through the incision or exudate from an infected incision. In these instances it is important to include absorptive cotton padding (such as a lined cotton roll) over the incision. An assistant holds the cotton in place while a second person begins by wrapping brown gauze around the horse's abdomen and handing it off to the first person. This is continued with 50% overlap of each wrap, using as many rolls of gauze as are needed to cover the padding material. The brown gauze is an optional layer, but does increase patient comfort during bandage changes by reducing the amount of hair that is pulled during bandage removal. (b) Once the brown gauze is applied the elastic tape is applied in a similar fashion, taking care to lay the tape half on the gauze and half on the hair to create a seal and help secure the bandage.

(c)

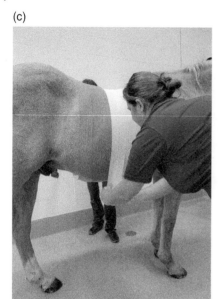

Figure 7.3 (Continued) (c) The elastic tape is circumferentially applied with ⅓–½ width overlap by passing the roll of tape between bandagers until the brown gauze is fully covered and a seal at the rear of the bandage is created. This will typically take three to five complete rolls of elastic tape. (d) If additional bandages are required, there is no need to fully remove the elastic tape. The tape can simply be cut adjacent to the padding on both sides of the horse.

(d)

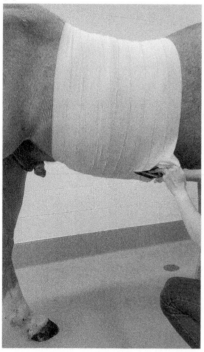

(e)

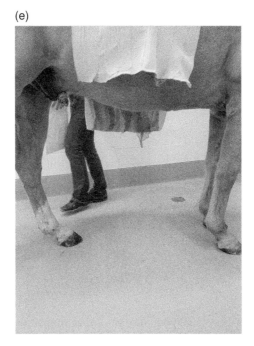

Figure 7.3 (Continued) (e) Once the ventral bandage is removed, any incisional care or wound treatment can be performed and the new bandage material applied ventrally, with the fresh elastic tape being applied directly over the initial layers. This method spares the horse from repeatedly having its hair pulled at every bandage change.

Table 7.2 Materials need for placement of an elastikon abdominal wrap bandage.

Material needed	Number
Combine cotton roll	1
Brown gauze	2–3 rolls
Elastikon	4–6 rolls

Section II

Application of Equine Limb Splints

8

Materials and Concepts for Splint Application

Splints are applied to equine limbs for either immobilization or support. The most important indication is for emergency stabilization of fractures or tendon/ligament ruptures. Other indications for splint application include wound/incision management in high-motion areas, to aid in the correction of flexural limb deformities, or to facilitate weight bearing in a horse with radial nerve paralysis. A key feature of these situations is that they all depend on appropriate application of the splints to be successful in managing the condition and in preventing injury to the horse.

The techniques demonstrated in this chapter are based on those commonly described in equine texts and review articles. Very little objective research has been performed to guide clinicians in selecting splinting techniques. Instead, clinicians rely on the combined experiences of generations of veterinarians taught in veterinary schools, passed down from mentors or colleagues, or sometimes through the school of hard knocks. Each clinician develops their own personal approach to these basic techniques. In some situations, specific splinting techniques have been developed and these are covered in the suggested reading list. Suffice it to say that no one approach is ideal for every indication or fracture.

Clinicians should base their splinting applications on their assessment of the limb and the forces they wish to neutralize with the splint. In a fracture situation, bending forces in two orthogonal planes as well as axial compression need to be addressed to appropriately stabilize a limb. In other situations, such as preventing dehiscence of a dorsal fetlock laceration repair, forces in only one plane (in this example, dorsal/palmar bending) need to be considered.

Equine Bandaging, Splinting, and Casting Techniques, First Edition. J Dylan Lutter, Haileigh Avellar, and Jen Panzer.
© 2024 John Wiley & Sons, Inc. Published 2024 by John Wiley & Sons, Inc.
Companion website: www.wiley.com/go/lutter/1e

Principles of Equine Limb Immobilization

Splinting for Wound Healing

The primary goal of splint application for wound/incision healing is to reduce or prevent motion of the wounded area and reduce the tension on the suture line if present. The applied splint should allow normal weight bearing of the limb, assuming the bones and supporting tendons/ligaments are intact. The splint should also be applied in a manner that facilitates practical removal and replacement for bandage changes and wound care.

The two most viable techniques to achieve these goals are bandage cast application or placing a splint on the dorsal or palmar/plantar surface of the limb. Bandage cast application will be covered in Chapter 13. In some situations it will be preferable to use a bandage cast whereas in others, due either to cost, practicality, or clinician preference, a splint will be chosen. Splints can be custom formed from cast material or fashioned from light yet rigid material such as PVC pipe or aluminum. Depending on the circumstances, wood or steel may also be a viable material choice. Splint bandage combinations represent a compromise between immobilization and wound management. These are not as rigid as a cast and in some instances placing a cast may be indicated or preferred (such as with flexor tendon lacerations). Specially designed splinting constructs have been created as an intermediate step to manage flexor tendon lacerations after cast removal but before complete removal of support.

To immobilize the limb distal to the carpus/tarsus, the splint should extend from the ground to the proximal metacarpus/metatarsus. In this region, splints are often placed on the palmar/plantar side of the limb and may be custom molded to the normal contour of the fetlock/pastern (Figure 8.1). Care must be taken to protect the soft tissues from rub sores and trauma induced by the splint, particularly the heel bulbs. The bandage may be placed sufficiently distal on the limb to accomplish this or padding may be added to the splint end for protection. If the splint is not custom molded to the limb, any space between the limb and splint should be filled with padding and incorporated into the bandage.

The carpus can be immobilized without affecting the fetlock and digits by extending a caudal splint from the proximal radius to the distal metacarpus, just proximal to the sesamoid bones (Figure 8.2). Most horses tolerate this very well and learn to walk without fighting the splint. In the hind limb, the reciprocal apparatus complicates splint placement. Cases of tarsal wounds that need immobilization are best managed using casts or bandage casts.

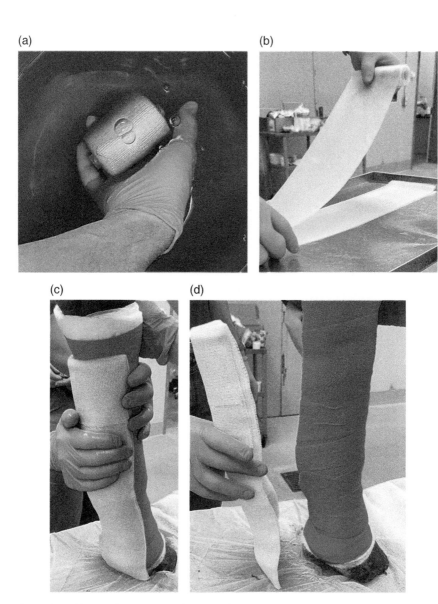

Figure 8.1 Process for custom molding a splint from fiberglass cast material.
(a) Submerse the cast material in warm water. To be sure the entire roll is fully wetted, it usually is best to keep it submerged until the bubbles have stopped escaping from the roll. (b) Either unroll the wet cast material onto a flat surface or hold it in hand with the help of an assistant. Fold it in a back-and-forth "accordion style" so that its length matches the required length on the limb to be splinted. More than one roll may be used, depending on the length and thickness desired. (c) Place the cast material onto the desired location of a pre-bandaged limb. Manually mold it to closely fit the contours of the limb, with an assistant's help if needed. Alternatively, a roll of cohesive bandage material may be used to secure the material to the limb. Pictured here is a half limb bandage used for splint molding. It is imperative that the limb not move during this process. Note that the heel bulbs are fully covered by the bandage to protect them from the cast material. (d) Once fully set and hardened, the cast material splint may be removed from the bandage, or it may be secured in place with an inelastic tape such as duct tape until a bandage change is required.

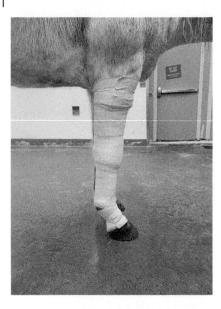

Figure 8.2 A carpal bandage cast has been placed on this patient to prevent carpal flexion and allow a dorsal carpal laceration to heal. This cast can be bivalved into cranial and caudal halves to allow for bandage changes with subsequent replacement of the clam-shelled cast splints. Alternatively, only one half of the cast splint may need to be used. Note that the cast material terminates proximal to the fetlock so as not to inhibit the motion of that joint.

Splinting for Flexural Deformities

Flexural deformities of the front limbs are a common reason for a neonatal foal to present for evaluation. Though such deformities are commonly called "contracted tendons," this is a misnomer as it is impossible for tendons to contract and it is usually not the tendons themselves that are the problem. In most cases the limb can be forced into a straight position to accommodate the placement of splints. Many of these foals can be successfully managed through the application of full limb palmar splints that span from the ground to the point of the elbow in addition to medical management. Foals should remain in stall confinement while the splints are in place.

Figure 8.3 shows the process of splint application. The foal should be sedated and restrained in lateral recumbency by two assistants. One assistant should be in control of the head and one in control of the hind limbs. A third assistant (if available) is assigned to handle bandage materials and assist in manipulating the limb being bandaged. The primary bandager's role is to ensure appropriate placement of the bandage and splint. The splints can remain in place for 12, 24, or even 48 hours, at clinician discretion, before removing and assessing the progress of limb straightening. The splints/bandage should be replaced immediately if the splints rotate to a location that is not directly caudal on the limb. Some cases may require multiple resets of the splints for several days in a row. As foals are weaned out of the splints, some contraction may recur. These foals may need to be managed with the splints on for 12 hours and off for 12 hours for several days before

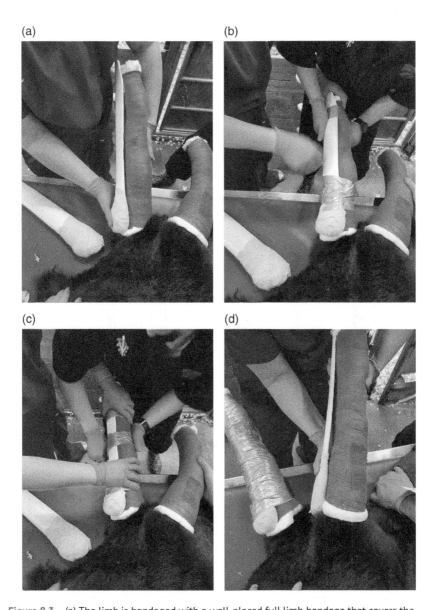

Figure 8.3 (a) The limb is bandaged with a well-placed full limb bandage that covers the soft tissues of the limb from the heel bulbs, proximally to the level of the elbow. Effectively, bandage material is placed as far proximal as is physically possible. The splint is placed palmarly/caudally and its length assessed so that the proximal end is at or near the point of the calcaneus. Cotton padding is added to the proximal end of the splint and secured with elastic tape to protect the soft tissues and prevent the development of sores. The distal end is situated so that the splint is in contact with the ground to bear the full weight of the foal. The foal's toe is positioned so that it is in contact with the ground but will not be in active weight bearing. (b) The splint is secured to the limb with one to two wraps of inelastic tape. Duct tape is used in this image. (c) The flexed fetlock and carpus are manually compressed to the splint and held in the straightened position by an assistant while the bandager applies the tape as tightly as possible, covering the entire leg. (d) The appearance of the fully splinted limb and positioning of a second splint on the contralateral limb. Note the gap that can be seen between the bandaged limb and the splint. This gap should be eliminated by the assistant manually compressing the limb to the splint during application of the tape.

finally discontinuing the splinting. In the most severely affected foals the flexural deformity is too extreme and the limb cannot be fully straightened to fit the splint. These severe cases may necessitate surgical tenotomy/desmotomy to correct the deformity.

Splinting for Limb Support and Fractures

The stakes of splinting a fractured limb are much higher than for wound management. Inappropriately stabilized fractures can damage fracture ends and surrounding soft tissues to the point that repair is impossible and euthanasia necessitated. The techniques demonstrated in subsequent chapters are examples of the current best practices for emergency field fracture stabilization. They were first reported by Bramlage in 1983 [1] and have been refined through continued use to successfully manage countless equine fracture patients. They have also been ineffectively applied to countless other patients, highlighting the importance of effective bandaging techniques and appropriate splint application.

It is important to realize that no single splinting technique is ideal for every fracture. Other techniques have been developed that are suitable or even preferable for specific fracture configurations. Readers are referred to the suggested reading at the end of the chapter for further information about these techniques.

Bandages for Splint Application

The importance of the bandage applied beneath the splints is an often-overlooked detail. A poorly applied bandage will allow excessive motion of a fracture and insufficient stabilization by the splints. This section provides context and explanation about recommendations previously made in the equine veterinary literature and texts.

Robert Jones Bandage

The Robert Jones bandage has historically been advocated for use in immobilizing the equine limb. This type of bandage was utilized by Sir Robert Jones, a Welsh surgeon in the late nineteenth and early twentieth centuries, and it came to bear his name. It was intended as a knee bandage to control swelling and has been used successfully by many physicians. Its adaptation to equine fracture management is classically described as using at least three layers of cotton padding <2 cm thick, each tightly bound by knitted or woven conforming material (such as brown gauze) and applied until the bandage diameter is three times that of the original limb. It relies on its mass/bulk as well as increasing tension being applied to each layer to aid in immobilization and overall bandage rigidity (Figure 8.4).

While some relatively stable or non-displaced fracture configurations may be supported by the Robert Jones bandage, the bandage alone is ineffective at immobilizing any unstable/displaced equine fracture. External splints must be secured to the bandage to provide the necessary rigidity and limb immobilization.

Modified Robert Jones Bandage

Many veterinarians refer to the use of a modified Robert Jones bandage. This generally means a similar style of bandage to the previously described Robert Jones bandage but with reduced bulk. This is often confusing to those unfamiliar with the term, because the amount of padding needed to make it modified (or not) is unspecified. Despite the persistent use of the term "Robert Jones," modified or not, to describe bandages applied with splints for equine field fracture stabilization, the majority of clinicians recognize that too much padding is detrimental to the stability of the bandage–splint construct. Generally, the term "modified Robert Jones" is used when the clinician wishes to convey that a stout bandage with substantial but not excessive padding was applied.

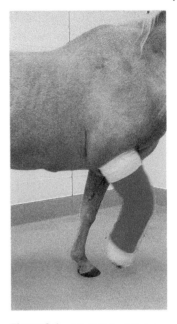

Figure 8.4 A full Robert Jones bandage has been applied to this horse's limb. The image demonstrates how much limb flexion is possible during ambulation following bandage placement. It highlights the importance of splint application for fracture stabilization, because a bandage alone does not immobilize the limb.

Evidence Base for Equine Fracture Splinting

Recently, several studies have experimentally investigated the effect of bandage technique (tension and padding) on sub-bandage pressure and the rigidity of various bandage–splint constructs. Canada et al. found that a single-layer distal limb bandage with cotton, brown gauze, and cohesive bandage maintained sub-bandage pressure for up to 96 hours after an initial pressure drop at the 6–12-hour mark [2]. In a subsequent paper they found that the single-layer distal limb bandage held significantly more sub-bandage pressure than a double-layer distal limb bandage that consisted of a cotton layer tightly bound by brown gauze, covered by another tight cotton–brown gauze layer, and finished with a covering of tightly applied cohesive bandage [3].

Lutter et al. investigated the effect of bandage material tension as well as the number of bandage layers on the resistance to bending of full limb bandage–splint constructs in a simulated fracture model [4]. They found that rigidity increased as the tension applied to the bandage material increased, but a threshold was reached when the tension applied to the material was roughly 94% of maximum. These authors also found that the rigidity of a single-layer full limb bandage, with external splints, was not significantly different than a three-layer Robert Jones–style full limb bandage with external splints. A pilot study for that paper found that Robert Jones bandages without splints applied completely failed in bending.

A subsequent study by Granello et al. [5] utilized cadaver limbs with an experimental transverse metacarpal III fracture. They investigated the sub-bandage pressure, radiographic alignment, and rigidity of the same bandage–splint constructs investigated by Lutter et al. Granello's findings support those of both Canada and Lutter, with the sub-bandage pressures being significantly higher in the single-layer bandage compared to the three-layer bandage, but no significant difference being found in bending. Interestingly, the fracture end alignment on radiographs was significantly better with the Robert Jones bandage–splint construct, implying that there may be a benefit to the increased padding despite the apparent lack of benefit in bandage rigidity.

The findings of these studies call into questions the theories used to justify the application of a Robert Jones–style bandage with splints for emergency equine fracture stabilization. More research into this area is needed to guide clinical techniques.

When bandaging for fracture stabilization, based on the evidence available, the authors recommend applying a single-layer bandage of appropriate height for splint application as tightly as possible (to the point of nearly ripping the material), with any gaps present between splint and bandage filled with padding and tightly bound to incorporate into the bandage. Splint selection and application are covered in the rest of this chapter and Chapters 9 and 10.

Splint Materials and Fabrication

The ideal splint material for emergency equine fracture stabilization is strong/rigid, lightweight, conforms to the leg or bandage, inexpensive, easily stored and transported, and readily applicable in a variety of situations.

While a variety of commercially produced splints are available, most can only be applied in a few situations and they can be relatively expensive. Some do not adequately stabilize the fractures for which they are designed. Others are constrained by the size of the horse they fit. Many are bulky and not conducive to easy storage in the veterinary truck. Given that equine fractures often occur at inopportune times in suboptimal environments, even the best splint is worthless if you don't have it with you. All of that said, these commercial splints are very useful when the right situation presents itself. Many veterinarians purchase one or two models to have on hand, should the need arise.

Fortunately, splints can be fashioned from a variety of commonly available materials, such as casting material, sectioned PVC pipe, wood (including boards or barn tool handles), conduit, metal rebar, and aluminum tubing or angle stock. Of these, PVC is the closest to being ideal. Schedule 40 PVC is white in color and most commonly available, but has a thinner wall thickness, whereas schedule 80 PVC is white or gray in color and has thicker walls. The type will be printed on the pipe. PVC pipe is inexpensive, available at any hardware store, and often is used at equestrian events for fences and obstacles. It can be easily heat molded and re-hardened, fashioned with hand tools, and (if sectioned pipe is used) stacked in a small pile and stored behind the truck seat or in a corner of the vet box. ABS is an alternative plastic pipe, black in color with similar properties to PVC, that may also be used.

Boards, such as 1×4 in. or 2×4 in., are preferred by some clinicians. Wood possesses many of the advantages of PVC, but is bulkier and not easily moldable in an urgent situation. One advantage of wood is that it can be fashioned into a heel wedge that may be useful in some situations.

PVC pipe of 4, 6, or 8 in. diameter can be cut into ½ or ⅓ circumference sections of the appropriate length, depending on the clinician's preference. One drawback of the 4 in. diameter is that the radius of the ½ section may be too tight to fit a bulky bandage and the radius of the ⅓ may not resist bending as well as desired. The radius of larger-diameter pipes may be so large that excessive padding needs to be added to assure a secure fit, potentially reducing the effectiveness of the splint. The authors prefer ⅓ sections of 6 in. pipe for its applicability to many situations, but have found that ⅓ sections of 4 in. pipe may be a better fit for a less bulky bandage.

Table 8.1 lists common splint lengths previously recommended for splinting specific fracture regions [6]. Preferred lengths will vary depending on the most common type/size of horse in a veterinarian's practice area. Splint lengths should be chosen and modified (if possible) based on each individual patient.

Splint fabrication can be as simple as cutting the selected material to the desired length and width with simple hand tools. However, having access to a workshop and knowledge of tools are helpful in fabricating, modifying, and customizing splints for each patient. Most refinements can be completed using a hand saw/hacksaw and sandpaper. Handheld power saws such as a circular saw or reciprocating saw will add speed to the process. A band saw or scroll saw is helpful for cutting custom shapes or curves.

Table 8.1 Common splint lengths and their corresponding region for use in an approximately 1000 lb (454 kg) horse.

Length	Limb region	Injuries splinted
14–16 in. (35–40 cm)	Splints extending to proximal metacarpus	Phalangeal fractures, fetlock sesamoid fractures, suspensory apparatus breakdown, tendon ruptures/lacerations
24–32 in. (60–80 cm)	Splints extending to the elbow and caudal olecranon	Metacarpal fractures, carpal fractures, olecranon fractures, possibly very distal radius fractures
55–60 in. (140–150 cm)	Lateral splints extending to the scapula or hip	Radius fractures, very distal humerus fractures
22–24 in. (55–60 cm)	Splints extending to the caudal calcaneus	Caudal splint for metatarsal fractures

A heat gun or torch is useful for molding PVC, but can easily burn the operator. Both PVC and ABS have maximum temperature tolerances of 180 °F and can be softened by submersing them in boiling water, which may be moderately safer than using a flame. Having a hose or bucket of cold water available is useful for quickly hardening a splint after shaping. Rounding the corners and rasping or sanding the edges of splints are useful details to add that reduce the pinch/rub spots on a splint, but are not necessarily a requirement for an effective splint. Heel wedges may be fabricated from 4–5 in. wooden posts and cut to length to fit under the horse's hoof when placed in a toe-touching position.

Fracture First Aid

Fracture first aid and initial stabilization of a fracture are challenging for any practitioner. Fractures tend to occur in suboptimal anatomic and geographic locations at all hours of the day. Often there is a distraught or frantic owner present and possibly law enforcement or members of the general public. Horses cannot ambulate well on only three legs and may be distressed themselves. This is an intimidating situation for anyone to walk into for which no amount of lecture or reading can fully prepare you.

When you encounter this situation remember the following:

- You are the animal healthcare expert. You get to dictate the assessment and care of the animal. People present at the scene may not be mentally or physically capable of handling the injured horse. One of the best decisions you can make is to assign a skilled and calm animal handler (i.e. your veterinary nurse or assistant) to assist you in assessing the animal.

- Human safety is of the utmost importance. Frequently, the attending veterinarian is looked toward as the person in charge. It is not worth any person being injured or killed for the sake of the horse. You should be aware of the actions and proximity of everyone involved so that safety is not jeopardized. Do not be afraid to emphatically dictate what others should do. This point is often ignored in the heat of the moment as passionate equine veterinarians, assistants, and equestrians work to help an injured horse. The authors are certainly guilty of putting themselves at risk for the sake of a horse and others despite knowing the dangers.

Full discussion of emergency field first aid is beyond the scope of this book, but it is helpful to consider certain aspects that go hand in hand with bandage and splint application. Selected medications and dosages are included in Table 8.2 for emergency reference. Table 8.3 is a list of supplies put together for a fracture kit that can be easily kept in a tote or duffel bag. The reader is directed to the suggested reading for further resources on equine emergency management.

The objectives of your initial assessment and stabilization are the following:

- Stop active bleeding.
- Stabilize the unstable fracture to:
  - Relieve patient pain and anxiety.
  - Protect vital soft tissue structures (vessels and nerves).
  - Prevent an open fracture from developing.
  - Preserve the integrity of the fracture fragment ends.
- Systemically assess the animal and develop a treatment plan.
- Determine the nature of the fracture.
- Provide appropriate wound care.
- Recommend/offer referral to an emergency hospital for further treatment.

Fracture Regions

Fractures of both the front and hind limbs of a horse can be grouped into four regions (Table 8.4), as originally described by Bramlage [1] and illustrated in Figure 8.5. Details regarding splint placement will be discussed in the region-specific sections of Chapters 9 and 10.

Table 8.2 Emergency first aid medications and supplies.

Supply/medication	Quantity/dosage	Common dose (1000 lb/ 454 kg horse)	Purpose
Xylazine hydrochloride 100 mg/ml	0.2–1 mg/kg	150–200 mg	Sedation/analgesia
Detomidine hydrochloride 10 mg/ml	0.01–0.02 mg/kg	3–5 mg	Sedation/analgesia
Butorphanol tartrate 10 mg/ml	0.01–0.1 mg/kg	5 mg – sedation 20–50 mg – analgesia	Sedation/analgesia
3 ml and 12 ml syringes	At least 6 each		Medication administration
18 ga 1.5 in. needles	At least 12		
Chlorhexidine or betadine scrub with gauze	Soaked gauze in scrub container		Skin antiseptic
2% or 4% chlorhexidine or 10% betadine solution	0.1–0.2% solution – betadine 0.025% solution – chlorhexidine		Wound lavage/ cleanse
70% Isopropyl alcohol with gauze	Soaked gauze in container		Skin cleanse and antiseptic
1 L bottles of 0.9% saline	1–2		Skin cleanse
Package of 4×4 in. gauze	1		
Clippers with #40 blade and blade spray	1; spare clipper blade		Hair clipping
IV catheter supplies: 14 ga 5 in. catheter, 2-0 suture, extension set, injection port cap, 10 drop IV set	1 each; consider spares		IV access
1 L and 5 L bags of lactated Ringer's or 0.9% saline	1–2 of each size		Wound lavage, IV fluid administration
Procaine penicillin G 300 000 IU/ml	22 000– 44 000 IU/kg IM q 12 h	35 ml	Infection prophylaxis
Gentamicin 100 mg/ml	6.6 mg/kg IV or IM q 24 h	30 ml	Infection prophylaxis

Table 8.2   (Continued)

Supply/medication	Quantity/dosage	Common dose (1000 lb/ 454 kg horse)	Purpose
Ceftiofur sodium 50 mg/ml	2.2 mg/kg IV or IM q 12 h	20 ml	Infection prophylaxis
Trimethoprim sulfa 960 mg tablets or powder	30 mg/kg PO q 12 h	14 tablets	Infection prophylaxis
Phenylbutazone 200 mg/ml, 1 g tablets	2.2–4.4 mg/kg q 12–24 h	1–2 tablets orally 10 ml injectable IV	Anti-inflammatory/ analgesic
Flunixin meglumine 50 mg/ ml or paste tubes	1.1 mg/kg IV or PO q 12 h	10 ml liquid or dose paste by weight	Anti-inflammatory/ analgesic

IM, intramuscularly; IV, intravenous; PO, orally; q, every.

Table 8.3   Supplies needed for a well-stocked equine fracture kit. The quantities listed here are more than may be used to successfully splint a fracture, but represent a sufficient number should more material be needed than is typically expected.

Supply	Quantity	Purpose
Telfa 3 × 4 in.	4	Primary layer; wound dressing
4 in. woven gauze roll (kling)	2	Secures telfa
16 in. cotton combine roll (CombiRoll) 20 in. (55 cm) length	4–6	Secondary layer; bandage padding
6 in. brown gauze roll	6 or pack of 12	Tertiary layer; binds and compresses cotton
4 in. cohesive bandage	6	Tertiary layer; compresses cotton, outer bandage layer
3 in. or 4 in. elastic tape	6 or two 4-packs	Seals bandage, secures padding in place
Duct tape or 2 in. athletic tape	2 rolls – duct tape 6–8 rolls – athletic tape	Secures splints in place
PVC splints, various lengths 4 in. or 6 in. diameter ⅓ section	2 each: 16 in., 30 in. 1 each: 36 in., 60 in.	Stabilizes fracture
Commercial splint, e.g. Kimzey Leg Saver	1	Stabilizes fracture

Table 8.4 Fracture regions of the equine limb with corresponding structures and splint placement.

Region	Structures supported	Splint placement
Forelimb		
I Distal limb	Phalanges and fetlock region fractures/ breakdown	Dorsal to proximal metacarpus Consider lateral splint if unstable
II Mid-limb	Metacarpal fractures, carpal fractures, distal metaphyseal radial fractures	Palmar/caudal to point of olecranon Lateral to level of elbow joint
III Forearm	Proximal and diaphyseal radial fractures, tibial fractures	Palmar/caudal to point of olecranon Lateral to level of scapula
IV Proximal limb	Olecranon, humeral, and distal scapular fractures	Consider palmar/caudal splint to level of olecranon for olecranon fracture; may not provide benefit in all horses with more proximal fractures Consider not splinting
Hind limb		
I Distal limb	Phalanges and fetlock region fractures/ breakdown	Plantar to point of calcaneus May consider dorsal placement Consider lateral splint if unstable
II Mid-limb	Metatarsal fractures, tarsal fractures and luxations	Plantar to point of calcaneus Lateral splint to level of calcaneus (metatarsal fractures) or stifle joint (tarsal fractures)
III Crus	Tibial fractures	Lateral splint to level of coxofemoral joint
IV Proximal limb	Femur and pelvic fractures	Cannot be splinted

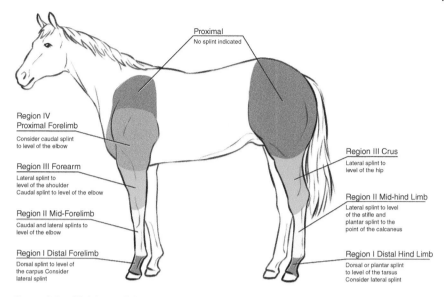

Figure 8.5 Divisions of the equine limb for splint application in the field stabilization of fractures.

References

1 Bramlage, L.R. (1983). Current concepts of first aid and transportation of the equine fracture patient. *Compend. Contin. Educ. Pract. Vet.* 5: S564–S573.

2 Canada, N.C., Beard, W.L., Guyan, M.E. et al. (2017). Measurement of distal limb sub-bandage pressure over 96 hours in horses. *Equine Vet. J.* 49 (3): 329–333.

3 Canada, N.C., Beard, W.L., Guyan, M.E. et al. (2018). Effect of bandaging techniques on sub-bandage pressures in the equine distal limb, carpus, and tarsus. *Vet. Surg.* 47: 640–647.

4 Lutter, J.D., Cary, J.A., Stephens, R.R. et al. (2015). Relative stiffness of 3 bandage/splint constructs for stabilization of equine midmetacarpal fractures. *J. Vet. Emerg. Crit. Care (San Antonio)* 25 (3): 379–387.

5 Granello, M.E., Weatherall, K.M., Lutter, J.D. et al. (2023). Comparison of two bandage splint constructs in an ex vivo equine metacarpal fracture model. *Vet. Comp. Orthop. Traumatol.* 36: 82–86.

6 Campell, N. (1996). Application of a Robert Jones bandage. In: *A Guide to the Management of Emergencies at Equine Competitions* (ed. S.J. Dyson), 21–28. Fordham: British Equine Veterinary Association.

Suggested Reading

Morgan, J.M. and Galuppo, L.D. (2021). Fracture stabilization and management in the field. *Vet. Clin. Equine.* 37: 293–309.

Wright, I.M. (2017). Racecourse fracture management. Part 1: Incidence and principles. *Equine Vet. Educ.* 29 (7): 391–400.

Wright, I.M. (2017). Racecourse fracture management. Part 2: Techniques for temporary immobilization and transport. *Equine Vet. Educ.* 29 (8): 440–451.

Wright, I.M. (2017). Racecourse fracture management. Part 3: Emergency care of specific fractures. *Equine Vet. Educ.* 29 (9): 500–515.

9

Distal Limb Splinting

Splinting of the distal limb is necessary in a variety of scenarios including managing wounds, soft tissue contracture, or for fracture first aid immobilization. This chapter will review the placement of PVC splints and a common commercially available splint.

Region I PVC Splinting – Phalanges and Distal Fetlock

Splinting for region I is applicable for fractures of the phalanges as well as suspensory breakdown injuries (Figure 9.1 and 9.2). Initial wound therapy should be considered prior to application of the bandage and splint. Under all scenarios when a splint needs to be utilized, a compression bandage needs to be placed. Refer to Chapter 2 for discussion on placement of a distal limb bandage. It is imperative that adequate padding is used to protect the limb from the splint and over any prominences, such as the heel bulbs.

The Kimzey splint is a well-known, commercially available splint device that has extensive utility for stabilization of severe injuries in the horse (Figure 9.3). This splint has many advantages, including a pre-contoured configuration and pre-placed wedge. Models are available without the built-in wedge. Velcro® straps allow for quick application. The company periodically updates models and changes the splint configuration. Clinicians should be aware of the pros and cons of each configuration for the types of fractures they are intended to stabilize. Modification of the splint after purchase, either at the manufacturer or at a local metal shop, may be necessary to achieve the desired configuration. The biggest disadvantage is that the Kimzey splint does not provide any medial to lateral support. In addition, some horses do not tolerate its placement and resort to kicking with their splinted leg, leading to a need for removal of the Kimzey.

Equine Bandaging, Splinting, and Casting Techniques, First Edition. J Dylan Lutter, Haileigh Avellar, and Jen Panzer.
© 2024 John Wiley & Sons, Inc. Published 2024 by John Wiley & Sons, Inc.
Companion website: www.wiley.com/go/lutter/1e

(a)

(b)

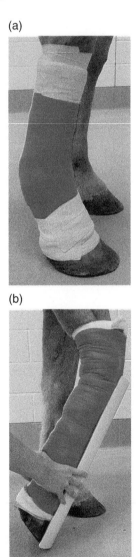

Figure 9.1 Application and proper placement of dorsal and lateral splints in the forelimb. (a) A distal limb compression bandage will be the starting point before application of any distal limb splint. Padding should be in place to fully cover the areas where the splints may contact. (b) The forelimb should be placed on the toe, aligning the dorsal bony column of the limb. The PVC should span from the ground at the toe to the carpo-metacarpal joint; the splint should be trimmed or altered if needed. It is important to place the splint on the midline for the most stable construct and ensure that it aligns with the longitudinal axis of the limb. Notice that additional bandage has been added to the proximal aspect of the bandage to protect the carpus from the splint. This has been placed in a routine fashion using cotton bound with brown gauze and fully compressed with cohesive bandage material.

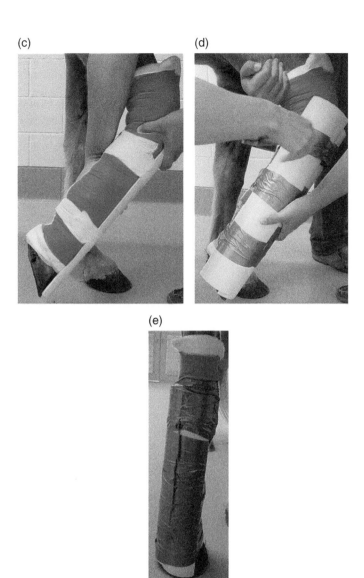

Figure 9.1 (Continued) (c) The dorsal splint is secured to the limb using non-elastic tape. Here, 2 in. porous athletic tape is being used. The authors prefer placing their initial tape at the proximal and distal ends for initial security. Depending on the injury, a dorsal splint may be all that is necessary for emergency coaptation. If this is the case, inelastic tape is wrapped from proximal to distal with 50% overlap until the bandage–splint construct is fully covered. If there is medial and lateral instability of the distal limb, a lateral splint may also be necessary. (d) If medial to lateral instability is appreciated or possible due to the nature of the fracture, a second splint should be placed on the lateral aspect of the limb from the ground to the carpo-metacarpal joint. The second splint is then secured to the limb using non-elastic tape such as duct tape or white athletic tape. (e) At the completion of splint placement non-elastic tape should be placed over the entirety of the construct, fully securing the splint material in place. Multiple layers can be used to add strength to the tape if a need is perceived. The splints should be held as tight as possible to the limb while being secured. Pay close attention that the splint remains in the correct orientation and does not slip from the midline. The horse should walk on its toe with no weight bearing on the heel.

(a) (b)

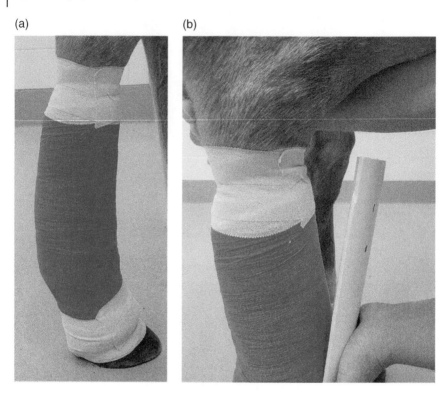

Figure 9.2 Application and proper placement of dorsal and lateral splints in the hind limb. Some texts will recommend plantar placement of the splint and extending the splint to the point of the calcaneus. Other authors have suggested wiring a board to the sole of the hoof, secured through the hoof wall, then flexing the fetlock to bring the board into contact with the plantar aspect of the limb and securing it with inelastic tape. The authors prefer the splint placement illustrated here, based on simplicity of application and their previous experience. Since none of these configurations have been evaluated objectively, it is ultimately up to each individual to decide which configuration to use. (a) Begin with a standard distal limb compression bandage. (b) The splint should be applied on the limb with the horse's distal bony column aligned and not bearing full weight. The splint should span from the ground to the proximal metatarsus. If the splint is too long or too short it should be modified. This image demonstrates a PVC splint that is too long and will rub the tarsus if placed in this manner. It will be trimmed to the proper length prior to application.

(c)

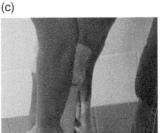
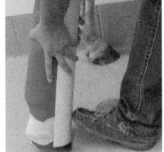

(d)

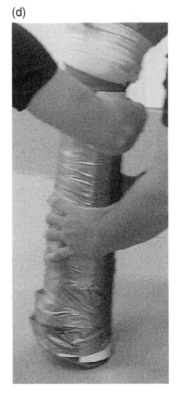

Figure 9.2 (Continued) (c) A properly measured dorsal splint is secured to the limb with non-elastic tape. It is important to ensure that the splint is on the midline and in line with the longitudinal axis of the limb to decrease the risk of rub sores and maximize stability. (d) A dorsal splint being secured with non-elastic tape. When placing the tape the splint should be held firmly to the leg and tape applied with as much tension as it will allow so that it is secured as tightly as possible. Pay close attention that the splint remains in the correct orientation and does not slip from the midline.

(e)   (f)   (g)

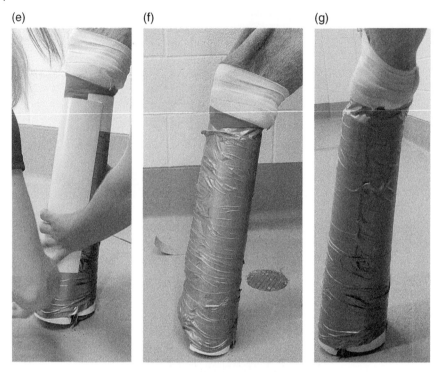

Figure 9.2 (Continued) (e) If medial to lateral instability is appreciated in the patient, an additional lateral splint should be applied in a similar manner as for the forelimb, from the ground to the proximal metatarsus, and secured with non-elastic tape. The overlap at the proximal end of the splints in this image will be corrected after the distal end is secured. (f) A lateral view of the finished bandage and splint application in the distal hind limb. (g) A dorsal view of the finished bandage and splint application in the distal hind limb.

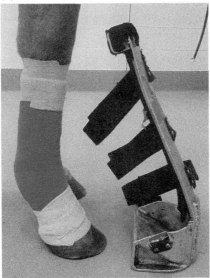

(a)

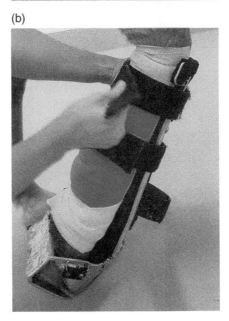

(b)

Figure 9.3 Application of a distal limb Kimzey leg saver splint in the forelimb or hind limb. Shown is an older splint model that has been modified with a heel wedge created to increase ground contact of the splint. Models without the heel wedge have been sold and recently the company has created a model which places the horse in a natural weight bearing position. (a) A standard half limb compression bandage should be placed to protect the limb from the splint. The splint does come fitted with neoprene foam padding that provides some protection, but the addition of a bandage to the limb allows the leg to conform better to the splint and enables the Velcro straps to be fitted more firmly. (b) The hoof of the affected limb is placed in the base of the splint, which forces the limb into alignment with the toe pointed. The Velcro straps are secured around the limb. Note that some horses may require flares to be trimmed from their hooves before they adequately fit into the splint. In addition, many larger horses have hooves that are too large to allow the use of the most common splint.

(c)

(d)

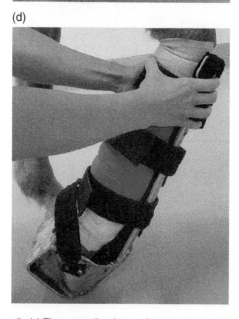

Figure 9.3 (Continued) (c) The most distal strap is secured around the heel bulbs and through the corresponding latch. This prevents the hoof from slipping out of the distal aspect of the splint. (d) After initial placement, all straps should be reset and tightened as securely as possible. If needed, the straps may be secured with tape to prevent them from becoming detached during transportation.

(e)

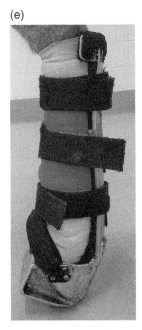

(f)

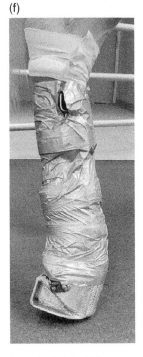

Figure 9.3 (Continued) (e) A view of a finished Kimzey splint applied to the forelimb. (f) The Kimzey splint can also be applied to a hind limb in the same fashion. A special splint is available for the hind limb with a more natural hoof position, but a forelimb splint can be used in an emergency scenario. When these splints have been utilized numerous times the Velcro may become compromised, so non-elastic tape may be used for additional security.

10

Full Limb Splinting

Splinting of the mid and upper limb may be necessary under emergency situations in which there are fractures of the metacarpus/metatarsus, carpus, radius, or tibia. This chapter will review the placement of PVC splints for regions II and III. Variations in the forelimb and hind limb will also be discussed.

Region II PVC Splinting – Metacarpus/Metatarsus and Carpus/Tarsus

Splinting for region II is applicable for fractures of the metacarpus, carpus, and distal metaphyseal radius in the forelimb (Figure 10.1), as well as fractures of the metatarsus and tarsus (Figure 10.2). Luxations of the tarsus should also utilize region II splinting techniques. Refer to Chapter 3 for discussion on placement of a full limb bandage. It is imperative that adequate padding is used to protect the limb from the splint and over any prominences, such as the heel bulbs, accessory carpal bone, and elbow.

Equine Bandaging, Splinting, and Casting Techniques, First Edition. J Dylan Lutter, Haileigh Avellar, and Jen Panzer.
© 2024 John Wiley & Sons, Inc. Published 2024 by John Wiley & Sons, Inc.
Companion website: www.wiley.com/go/lutter/1e

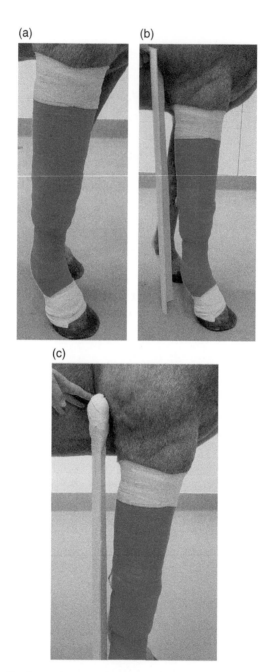

Figure 10.1 Application and proper placement of a caudal and lateral splint in the forelimb for region II. (a) A full limb compression bandage will be the starting point before application of any distal limb splint. Padding should be in place to fully cover the areas where the splints may contact. (b) The caudal splint should be measured next to the horse prior to any trimming. The splint should fully span from the ground to the point of the elbow (olecranon). After measurements have been made, the edges of the splint should be rounded and padded. (c) Rolled cotton or CombiRoll may be used to give the splint additional padding at the most proximal and distal aspects. This padding may be secured with non-elastic or elastic tape.

(d)

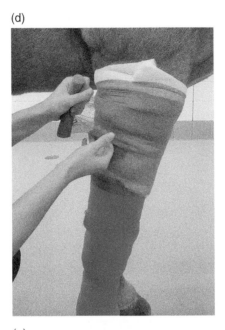

(e)

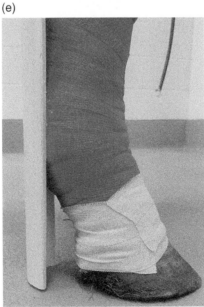

Figure 10.1 (Continued) (d) The limb should also include bandaging as far proximal as possible to decrease the risk of splint sores over any bony prominence. Partial rolls of combi-cotton can be used to achieve this. Three layers of bandage should be placed (cotton, brown gauze, and vet wrap). (e) Due to the angle at the fetlock, there is usually space between the splint and the pastern. To decrease the stress of the splint at this location, additional padding can be added to decrease this space.

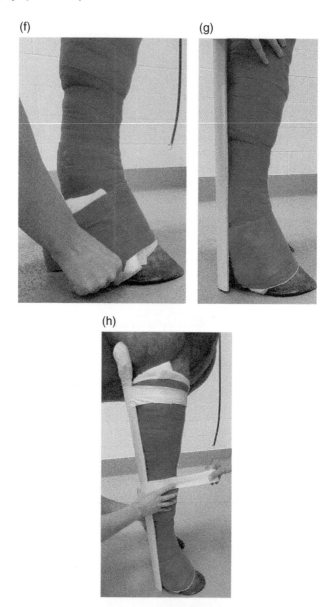

Figure 10.1 (Continued) (f) A stack of gauze or additional combi-cotton can be placed at the palmar pastern and secured with vet wrap. (g) The palmar splint lays flush with the bandaged limb. (h) The caudal splint is secured from the ground to the point of the elbow directly on the midline using non-elastic tape. Here, 2 in. porous athletic tape is being used. The authors prefer placing their initial tape at the proximal, middle, and distal ends for initial security.

Figure 10.1 (Continued) (i) A view of the caudal splint from the caudal aspect of the limb. Note the midline placement of the splint with no medial or lateral deviation. Additional padding may be placed at the elbow following full splint application. (j) The lateral splint is measured and should span from the ground to the proximal radius. The proximal and distal aspects of the splint may need to be rounded or padded further if excessive pressure is placed on the limb, to prevent splint sores. In the case shown the bandage is acting with adequate padding for emergency coaptation; if long-term immobilization is needed additional splint contouring should be considered. (k) The lateral splint continues to be secured to the limb with non-elastic tape in multiple locations. The splint should be placed flat to the lateral aspect of the limb with very little open space between the bandage and the splint. (l) A dorsal view of the lateral and caudal splint placement. Notice the gaps present between the lateral splint and the bandaged limb. Ideally, these gaps would be filled with additional padding to increase contact between the splint and the leg and improve alignment of the fracture ends.

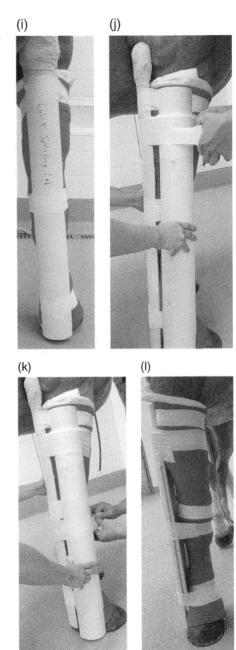

(m) (n)

(o)

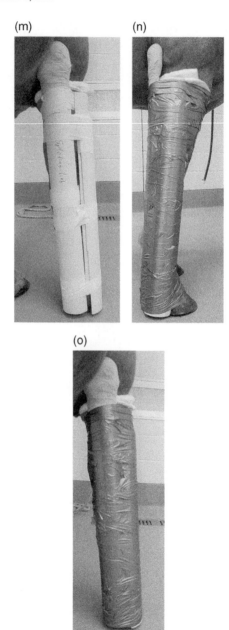

Figure 10.1 (Continued) (m) A caudal view of the lateral and caudal splint placement. (n) At the completion of splint placement, non-elastic tape should be placed over the entirety of the construct, fully securing the splint material in place. Multiple layers can be used to add strength to the tape if a need is perceived. The splints should be held as tight as possible to the limb while being secured. Pay close attention that the splint remains in the correct orientation and does not slip from the midline. (o) A caudal view of the completed splint complex. Note the midline placement of the caudal splint.

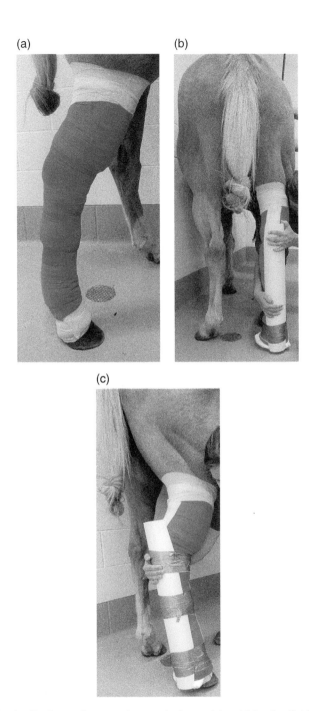

Figure 10.2 Application and proper placement of a caudal and lateral splint in the hind limb for region II. (a) A splint for region II in the hind limb begins with a standard full limb compression bandage. Padding should be in place to fully cover the areas where the splints may contact. (b) The caudal splint is typically placed first. The splint should be measured and span from the ground to the point of the calcaneus. Due to the angle of the hock in the hind limb, longer caudal splints do not provide any additional stability to the construct. It is imperative the splint is placed directly on the midline and does not deviate medially or laterally. (c) The caudal splint can be secured by non-elastic tape in several locations.

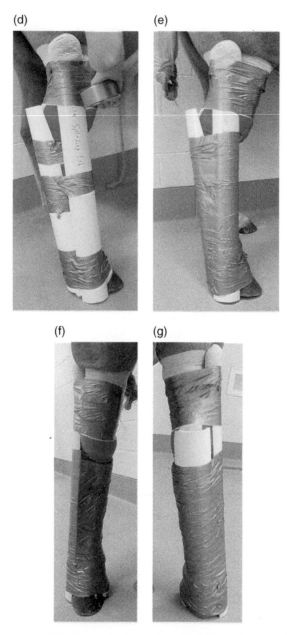

Figure 10.2 (Continued) (d) A lateral splint is then placed from the ground to the level of the stifle. It is important to ensure that the proximal aspect of the splint is properly padded if it sits above the level of the bandage. The lateral splint is once again secured to the limb using non-elastic tape. (e) A lateral view of a completed splint–bandage complex for region II of the hind limb. (f) A dorsal view of a completed splint–bandage complex for region II of the hind limb. (g) A caudal view of a completed splint–bandage complex for region II of the hind limb.

Region III PVC Splinting – Radius, Ulna, and Tibia

Splinting for region III is applicable for fractures of the proximal and diaphyseal region of the radius in the forelimb (Figure 10.3) and fractures of the tibia in the hind limb (Figure 10.4). Due to the large muscle mass in the upper limbs of horses, fixation of the elbow and stifle is difficult. Risk of skin penetration of fracture ends can occur with abduction of the limb; for this reason full-length lateral splints are recommended.

In addition, radial nerve injuries or fractures of the ulna require splinting of the forelimb to assist in weight bearing and healing. Both of these injuries result in failure of the triceps muscles and passive stay apparatus of the forelimb, leading to the horse being unable to bear weight on the limb. Radial nerve injuries can occur without a fracture. Management of radial nerve paralysis and ulnar fractures cases is also touched on in Figure 10.3.

Refer to Chapter 3 for discussion on placement of a full limb bandage.

(a)   (b)   (c)

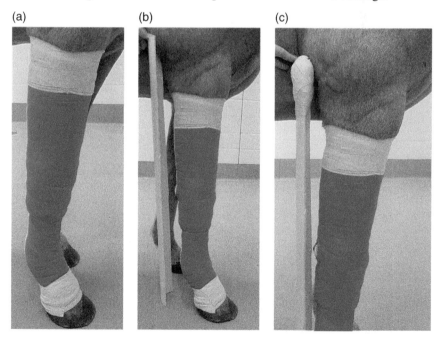

Figure 10.3 Application of caudal and lateral splints for region III of the forelimb. For horses experiencing radial nerve paralysis and ulnar fractures follow steps a–l, as only placement of a caudal splint is necessary. Patients with radial fractures require both caudal and full lateral splints for adequate immobilization. (a) A full limb compression bandage will be the starting point before application of any distal limb splint. Padding should be in place to fully cover the areas where the splints may contact. (b) The caudal splint should be measured next to the horse prior to any trimming. The splint should fully span from the ground to the point of the elbow (olecranon). After measurements have been made, the edges of the splint should be rounded and padded. (c) Rolled cotton or CombiRoll may be used to give the splint additional padding at the most proximal and distal aspects. This padding may be secured with non-elastic or elastic tape.

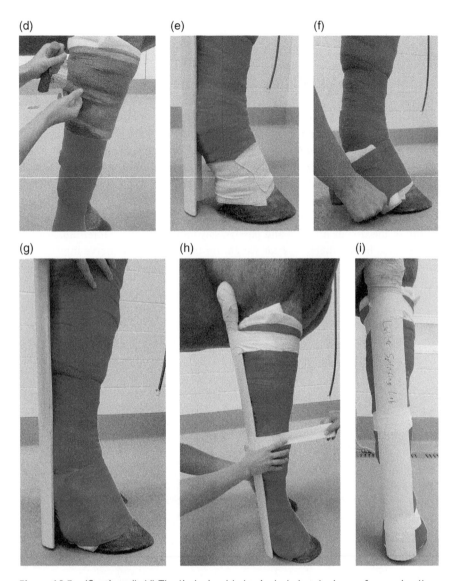

Figure 10.3 (Continued) (d) The limb should also include bandaging as far proximally as possible to decrease the risk of splint sores over any bony prominence. Partial rolls of combi-cotton can be used to achieve this. Three layers of bandage should be placed (cotton, brown gauze, and vet wrap). (e) Due to the angle at the fetlock, there is usually space between the splint and the pastern. To decrease stress on the splint at this location, additional padding can be added to decrease this space. (f) A stack of gauze or additional combi-cotton can be placed at the palmar pastern and secured with vet wrap. (g) The palmar splint lays flush with the caudal aspect of the bandaged limb. (h) The caudal splint is secured from the ground to the point of the elbow directly on the midline using non-elastic tape. Here, 2 in. porous athletic tape is being used. The authors prefer placing their initial tape at the proximal, middle, and distal ends for initial security. (i) A view of the caudal splint from the caudal aspect of the limb. Note the midline placement of the splint with no medial or lateral deviation. Additional padding may be placed at the elbow following full splint application. For horses experiencing radial nerve paralysis (no fracture), the splint can be fully secured to the bandage with non-elastic tape spanning the entire length of the limb. For horses experiencing fractures of the radius, the subsequent steps should be followed.

(j)   (k)

(l)   (m)

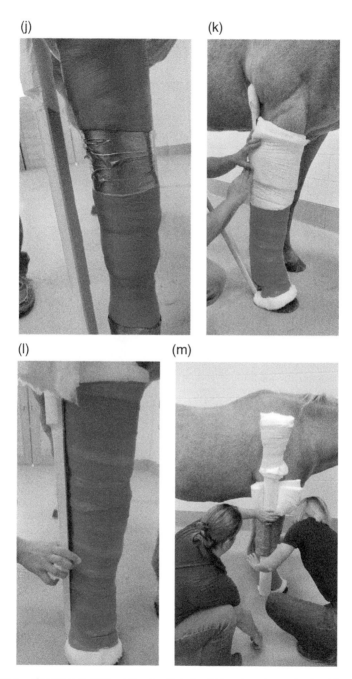

Figure 10.3   (Continued) (j) The lateral splint should be placed next. It should span from the ground to the proximal scapula. If the splint does not lay flush to the limb (as in this image), more padding should be added to the bandage. (k) A demonstration of additional cotton combi-roll being added to the bandage to allow the lateral splint to lay flush to the bandaged limb. (l) The full limb lateral splint now lays flush to the bandage and is ready to secure to the limb. (m) The full length lateral splint is secured to the limb using non-elastic tape. Note the additional padding on the proximal forelimb where bandaging is not easily performed.

(n)

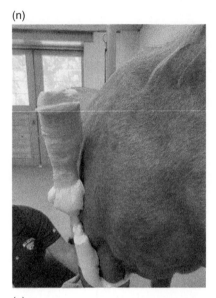

(o)

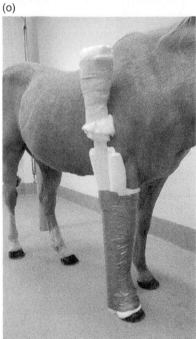

Figure 10.3 (Continued) (n) The proximal aspect of the lateral splint should be covered with additional padding if there is any risk of causing any cutaneous trauma to the horse. This can be done with cotton material secured with tape. (o) A craniolateral view of the completed region III splinting in the forelimb.

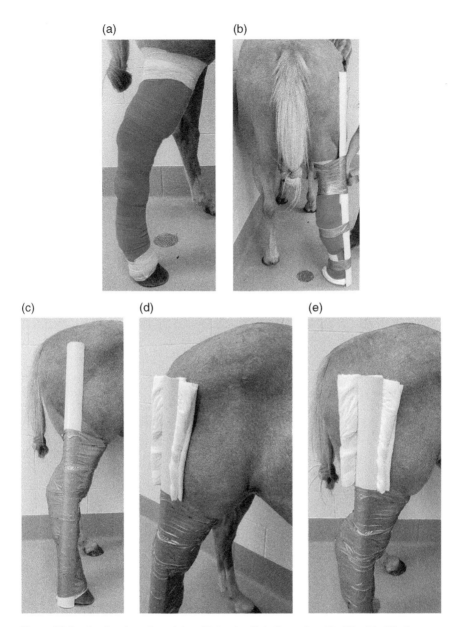

Figure 10.4 Application of caudal and lateral splints for region III of the hind limb. (a) A splint for region III in the hind limb begins with a standard full limb compression bandage. Padding should be in place to fully cover the areas where the splints may contact. (b) The splint should be placed laterally from the ground to the level of the tuber coxae and secured in multiple locations using non-elastic tape. If there is any open space between the bandaged limb and the splint, more padding should be added to allow direct contact between splint and limb. Note the direct contact of the splint in this case. (c) The splint should be secured to the bandaged limb using multiple layers of non-elastic tape. Note the alignment of the limb. The goal of the lateral splint is to prevent abduction and potential skin penetration by the fracture ends. (d) Additional padding between the proximal musculature and the splint is recommended to prevent any cutaneous trauma from the splint. Ideally, this padding should be secured to the splint to prevent its slippage during ambulation and transportation. (e) A different perspective of the proximal splint in relation to the limb with padding added to prevent abrasions from the splint.

Section III

Application of Equine Casts

11

Materials and Concepts for Cast Application

Casts are applied to equine limbs for similar reasons to splint application. Often casts are elected as a means of longer-term (days to weeks or months) limb immobilization or support compared to the usual short-term application of splints (hours to a few weeks). Most commonly casts are applied for stabilization of distal limb fractures, joint luxations, tendon lacerations, or wounds in high-motion areas, but they also are applied for additional protection of fracture repairs during and after anesthetic recovery.

There are four types of casts that may be applied to the equine limb: conventional casts, bandage casts, tube casts, and transfixation pin casts. Bandage casts will be covered in Chapter 13. Chapters 12, 14, and 15 will focus on the application of conventional casts.

Tube casts, sometimes called sleeve casts (Figure 11.1), are usually only used to stabilize foals with angular limb deformities due to incomplete ossification of cuboidal bones, or in orthopedic cases where either complete or partial carpal arthrodesis is indicated. The principles discussed for conventional casts are applicable for tube casts, with the exception that the distal aspect of the cast stops before it reaches the fetlock and the foot remains in contact with the ground.

Transfixation pin casts are useful for the management of severely comminuted fractures where fracture reconstruction with internal fixation is not possible, or in some situations with more simple fractures where financial constraints limit treatment options (Figure 11.2). After aseptic pin placement through the indicated bone proximal to the fracture, a conventional cast is applied that incorporates the pins and envelops the entire limb and foot distal to the fracture. The cast becomes the weight-bearing structure and transfers the force to the pins. The fractured limb essentially floats inside the cast without bearing a load. Specific principles should be followed for placement of the pins that are beyond the scope of this book.

Equine Bandaging, Splinting, and Casting Techniques, First Edition. J Dylan Lutter, Haileigh Avellar, and Jen Panzer.
© 2024 John Wiley & Sons, Inc. Published 2024 by John Wiley & Sons, Inc.
Companion website: www.wiley.com/go/lutter/1e

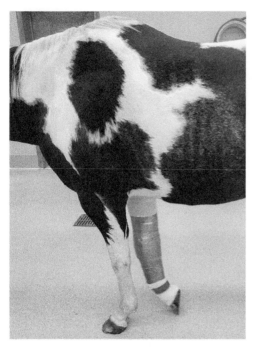

Figure 11.1 A tube cast has been applied to this patient in the form of a bandage cast to immobilize a severe carpal laceration. The bandage cast was required because the laceration required daily wound care and the tube cast was employed to allow mobility of the distal limb and ease the ambulation of the patient. Notice how the horse drags its toe during ambulation as a result of the carpus being locked in extension. The cast has been "bivalved" or "clam shelled" into cranial and caudal halves to facilitate bandage changes and then re-secured with duct tape.

(a)

(b)

(c)

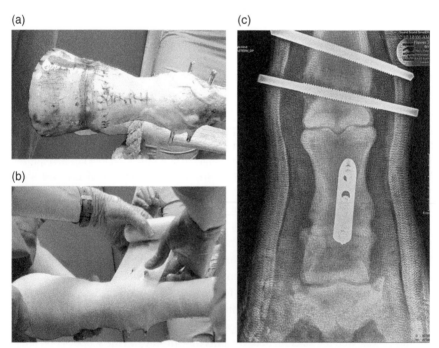

Figure 11.2 (a) The patient sustained a severely comminuted fracture of the second phalanx that is being managed with a transfixation pin cast. The image depicts a cast change under anesthesia and shows the 6.3 mm pins that were placed through the distal metaphysis of the third metatarsal bone. (b) The cast material is being applied to incorporate the pins. (c) This radiograph, taken eight weeks post-operatively, shows the pin placement through the third metatarsal bone and illustrates how the distal limb is suspended inside the cast.

Readers should refer to the suggested reading for more information on the use of these specialized casts and the procedures in which they are used.

Casting Team

Prior to beginning cast application, it is important to determine who will be assisting in the procedure and what roles they will fill. Because cast application is a time-sensitive procedure, it is important that all involved individuals know what will be occurring and what might be needed throughout, either routinely or as a contingency. The larger and more complex the cast, the more people need to be involved to ensure the application goes smoothly. If necessary, two people can place a simple cast if there is no one else available, but the entire procedure will go more smoothly if at least three people are present and dedicated to the cast application: the primary cast applicator, the primary cast material handler, and an assistant.

The cast applicator is generally the clinician in charge of the case and often, but not always, is the most experienced member of the group. Their role is to ensure that cast materials are applied in the proper sequence, to direct the material handler when to submerge the next roll, and ultimately to ensure that the cast material itself is applied correctly.

The cast material handler is usually the veterinary technician assigned to the case or casting procedure, but may be another veterinarian who is assisting. Often this person knows the preferences and expectations of the clinician in charge and frequently is very experienced in cast application. In addition to preparing the cast materials prior to application and submerging the cast material rolls, the material handler's role is to help direct the remainder of the team while the applicator is focused on the procedure and applying the cast materials. They should think ahead about what is needed, and what might happen, and prepare supplies that may be needed should things go wrong. Preparing more materials than are expected to be needed is an important part of the thought process for this team member.

At least one additional assistant is preferred to help the casting procedure proceed smoothly. This person's role is to be present and aware of what is happening and to assist as directed by the cast applicator. Two common things that are needed during cast application are the ready use of good-quality bandage scissors and being available to apply water to the cast material should it not be sufficiently wetted. Additional assistants can be very helpful, especially during difficult or very involved casting procedures. These individuals can assist in positioning the leg and ensure it remains still, serve as an additional material handler, or simply help with restraint of the horse if the cast is being applied in a standing position.

Patient Preparation for Cast Application

All wounds and surgical sites should be clipped and prepped routinely as their care dictates. Prior to cast application these sites should be dressed according to clinician discretion. As much hair as possible should remain on the leg to provide additional protection from cast sores. Sites that are predisposed to developing cast sores can have additional materials placed for added protection. A light inner bandage, as shown in Figure 1.5, can be applied to the limb with elastic tape where the tape can act as a second skin layer to protect against sores. Additionally, the authors have used the hydrogel bandage dressing Tegaderm™ by 3M in areas prone to developing rub sores. Dorsally at the proximal edge of the cast, at the base of the fetlock, and at the palmar aspect of the heel bulbs are all areas where cast sores commonly develop.

The shoe should be pulled prior to cast application. The hoof should be cleaned of gross debris, trimmed if needed, and an antiseptic such as tincture of iodine or Kopertox® applied to the frog sulci to prevent thrush development.

Limb Positioning for Cast Application

The cast can be applied with the horse standing in some cases, as long as the horse can be sufficiently sedated and remain still throughout the cast application and curing. The limb may be held in a raised position or the horse can be stood on blocks with the heels overhanging the edge, so that the cast material can be wrapped underneath them. This locks the heels and foot in position so that after it has cured the limb may be picked up and the hoof capsule fully enclosed with cast material (Figure 11.3).

Hind limbs in particular can be difficult to cast in a standing position because of the reciprocal apparatus and often require the horse to be anesthetized in lateral recumbency. Regardless of standing or anesthetized application, it is important the limb be placed in as normal a weight-bearing position as possible to increase the comfort of the horse and reduce the incidence of cast sores.

Some conditions, such as a flexor tendon laceration, benefit from positioning the limb in a toe-touching position with the dorsal cortices of the phalanges and metacarpus/ metatarsus aligned. Some clinicians prefer to use this positioning exclusively.

Cast Materials and Method of Application

The materials of a cast consist of the stockinette, cast padding, orthopedic felt, and fiberglass cast tape. The exact details of applying each layer will be covered in the individual cast chapters. Details of preparing the materials and, where helpful, a brief description of their application are covered here.

(a)

(b)

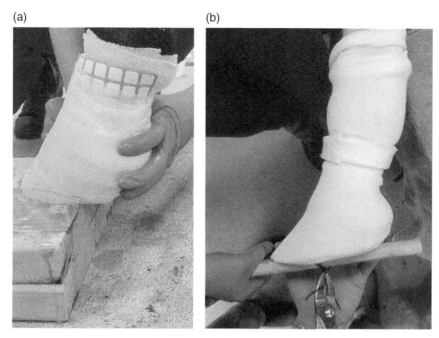

Figure 11.3 Examples of positioning a horse's limb for cast application. (a) Here the patient is stood bilaterally on blocks with the heels over the edge and the cast material is being wrapped underneath the heels to lock them in place. (b) In this image a phalangeal cast is being placed with the horse under anesthesia. A cut-off twitch handle is being wired to the hoof to steady it and maintain it in a normal weight-bearing position.

Stockinette

Stockinette should be applied in a double layer and cut sufficiently longer than the intended cast length by several inches. It may be omitted in some instances with certain cast padding materials where the cast is intended to become wet, but in general the authors recommend its use as an additional protective layer.

To prepare the stockinette, a length more than double the planned cast length and of sufficient diameter to fit over the foot is cut. Stockinette of 3 in., 4 in., or 6 in. diameter is common in horses. Each end is rolled toward the mid-point of the stockinette, with one end being rolled out and the other end being rolled in. This rolling continues until the ends meet in the middle. A twist is then applied on the stockinette and it is ready for application. Figure 11.4 demonstrates how each end is rolled. Typically, after stockinette application orthopedic felt is taped in place circumferentially on the leg at the intended location of the proximal aspect of the cast as well as overlying the heel bulbs.

(a)   (b)

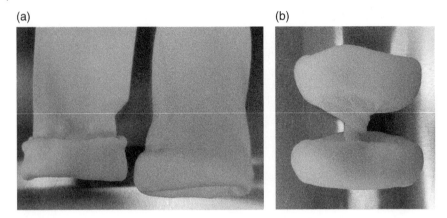

Figure 11.4   (a) The length of stockinette is rolled to apply a double layer directly on the limb. One end is rolled outward (the left-hand roll) and the other end is rolled inward (the right-hand roll). (b) Once the two ends meet in the middle, a twist is applied to the stockinette and it is ready for application to the leg.

Cast Padding

Cast padding should be applied regardless of the use of stockinette. Its purpose is to protect the leg from compression and abrasion by the rigid woven fiberglass cast tape. There is no guideline for the amount of cast padding that should be used, but the smallest amount that will sufficiently protect the skin should be the goal. Excessive cast padding will create a looser cast and promote movement of the limb within, which promotes cast sores and destabilizes the structure the cast is intending to stabilize.

Thin cast padding such as thin rayon/cotton rolls, sold as specialist cast padding, requires more layers of padding, whereas thicker synthetic materials such as Gore Procel® cast liner or Delta-Dry® cast padding require only a single layer applied with 50% overlap. Figure 11.5 illustrates these three types of cast padding.

Obstetric wires threaded through intravenous tubing, cut sufficiently longer than the cast, and placed on the medial and lateral sides of the cast can be utilized after cast padding but prior to application of the casting tape to facilitate cast removal without the use of an oscillating saw. If this is done it is important to cut the wire sufficiently long so that it can be grasped at the time of cast removal. The excess wire is taped out of the way during cast application. The ends are then coiled, held on the cast itself, and covered with elastic tape after the cast has fully cured in order to secure them in place for the duration of casting.

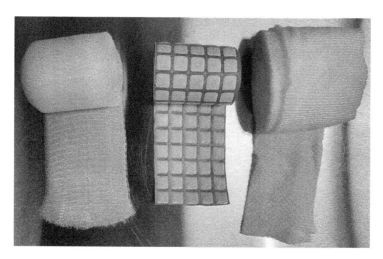

Figure 11.5 Delta-Dry (left) is a water-resistant knit cast padding commonly used in the authors' clinic. It retains its compressibility and is not deformed over time within the cast. It conforms well to the limb as it is applied. The main drawbacks are that it is not inexpensive and it firmly adheres to the cast tape, so it can make standing cast removal difficult. Gore Procel cast liner (middle) is made up of square cells containing polytetrafluoroethylene foam, which is a water-resistant and highly effective cast padding. One side of the Procel has a slight adhesive applied to help it remain in place after application. The only drawback of this material is that it does not easily conform to the leg during application and wrinkles or unintended overlaps are common. This does not appear to negatively affect its function or promote cast sores. It also does not appear to adhere as firmly to the cast tape, so removal may be less difficult compared to the Delta-Dry. Specialist cast padding (right) is a rayon/cotton fiber blend that is inexpensive, easily applied, and conforms well to the leg. The primary downside of this material is that it becomes compressed over time, allowing motion within the cast, and is not water resistant, so it must be kept dry. Specialist cast padding is very easily torn.

Cast Tape

Historically, plaster of Paris cast tape was used before the development of resin-impregnated fiberglass cast material. While it is still available for purchase, it has largely been replaced by fiberglass cast tape due to the latter's superior water resistance, improved breathability, lighter weight, and faster curing times. Numerous brands of various widths, resin characteristics, and fiberglass colors are available.

In general, the widest tape that can be conformed to the leg with the fewest number of wrinkles should be used so that the layers of cast tape have improved bonding capability. It may be helpful to start with a single narrow roll and move to wider rolls for subsequent layers. The authors' preferences for width will be listed at the beginning of each chapter.

(a)

(b)

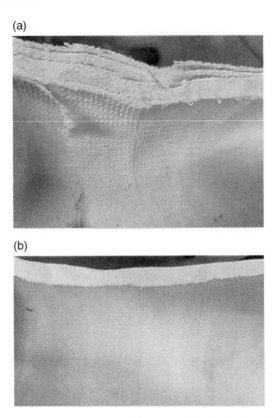

Figure 11.6 (a) This section of cast material was not fully bonded together and is substantially weaker than a fully bonded portion. Notice the delamination of the cast material. This could be caused by expired cast material, using material that was not fully wetted, or applying the material after the resin had set. (b) This section of cast material is fully bonded together, forming a strong, thick cast.

The resin impregnated in the fiberglass is water and temperature (heat) activated. Hardened, dry, or expired cast tape should not be used, as the layers will not bond together and will result in a weakened cast that is prone to breaking (Figure 11.6).

Each brand manufacturer will have specific water temperature, submersion time, and squeezing recommendations. Each roll of cast tape should be submerged in water that is between room temperature and bath water temperature, preferably closer to the latter. Between 3 L and 5 L of water should be sufficient for a half limb cast, but it is never wrong to prepare extra water. If given the choice, the authors prefer not to squeeze the cast roll, but this is clinician and cast material dependent. If the roll is not submerged long enough the inner layers will not become wet and activated, but if it is submerged too long the resin will begin to set before application to the leg. A good rule of thumb for most brands of cast material is to watch the bubbles coming from the submerged roll. Once the bubbles stop, the roll is ready to apply. It may be helpful to practice with your chosen brand to know how it is best handled.

The cast applicator should start the first roll at the top of the cast over the orthopedic felt and take an initial wrap around the leg to secure the tape, and then should proceed to wrap distally with 50% overlap of the width of the cast tape while applying minimal tension. The tension should not be enough to compress the cast padding, but should be sufficient to promote smooth application of the cast tape without forming wrinkles.

The speed of the cast applicator and the temperature of the water will determine the timing for an assistant to dunk the next roll of cast tape. It is the applicator's role to inform the assistant when to do this, but the assistant should feel empowered to ask when to submerge or even dunk the roll unprompted if the assistant has sufficient experience to judge the timing. In general, with an experienced team, the subsequent roll of cast tape can be submerged as soon as the previous roll is handed to the cast applicator. Each sequential roll of cast tape should begin where the previous roll ended so as not to create an area that is too thick and another area that is too thin. The number of rolls of cast tape used will depend on the width, but in general at least five to six layers of cast tape should be applied to the limb; more can be planned if added strength is desired.

Further techniques for strengthening the cast can be employed, such as adding an accordion-folded cast material splint within the cast. This and other techniques are more advanced, require more coordinated assistants, and should not be attempted until at least one member of the team is sufficiently experienced in cast application.

It is not uncommon for cast tape rolls following the first one not to be fully wetted before the applicator is ready for them. In those situations the roll should be handed to the applicator to avoid a delay in application and a water scoop be used to apply water to the cast tape as it is being applied, at the direction of the cast applicator. Usually, it is the inner third of the roll that is not sufficiently wetted. Proper preparation should ensure that a water cup is available and ready. If needed, the cast tape package wrapper makes for a convenient water scoop in these situations, particularly if the assistant only tears the edge of the wrapper.

Once sufficient layers have been applied, the cast should be gently rubbed to promote bonding of the layers until the resin begins to harden. Once that begins the cast can be left to fully cure over the next several minutes. The methods shown in later chapters leave the toe of the hoof exposed. Once the initial cast material has cured, a final roll of cast material is applied to fully enclose the foot.

After the cast has cured, an acrylic such as Technovit®, or an epoxy such as Super-Fast™ or Bovi-Bond, should be applied to the bottom of the cast to prevent premature wearing of the cast as the patient walks. The authors prefer to use acrylic because it can be molded during hardening to a shaped ground contact surface to facilitate patient mobility, but this material does add several minutes to the procedure for the curing time. Refer to later chapters for images and descriptions of the process for applying the acrylic to a cast.

A downside of acrylic is that it becomes so hard that it is slippery when the patient is walking on a concrete surface. This can be mitigated by wrapping the cured acrylic with elastic tape to increase the grip and replacing the tape as it becomes worn.

Finally, the top of the cast should be sealed with elastic tape, similar to a bandage, where one to two wraps of tape are applied with half of the tape on the cast and half on the skin.

Cast Management and Complications

Horses with a casted limb should be kept in a clean, dry, confined space and monitored closely for the duration of casting. The contralateral foot should be placed in a cushioned support boot, such as a Soft-Ride boot, or shod as the clinician desires to improve foot support and equalize the height with the casted limb. The duration of casting depends on the condition being treated and the conditions where the horse is kept. It can be as short as a few hours for emergency fracture stabilization prior to internal fixation, or as long as four to six weeks for managing flexor tendon lacerations. Most commonly, a cast is maintained for approximately two weeks before a cast change occurs and the limb is examined/treated. Then the decision for placing a second cast is made. In many instances a second cast is planned from the outset and already prepared at the beginning of removal of the first cast.

At a minimum the cast should be physically examined twice daily for cleanliness, moisture, and signs of developing problems underneath. The cast should remain clean and dry at all times. Every 24–48 hours the elastic tape at the top of the cast should be changed to ensure the top stays sealed, preventing debris from entering the cast, and to monitor for cast sore development at the top of the cast. Moisture may be felt on the cast surface if wound exudate accumulates underneath and seeps to the surface. Often the first sign this is occurring is the appearance of a stain on the cast or adherence of stall shavings on a particular problem area. If these signs go unnoticed, then secondary signs include lameness or reluctance to use the leg and finally the appearance of actual purulent exudate. Once the exudate is visible, there are often multiple other signs of problems and the state of the limb within the cast may be severely compromised.

Assuming the reason for casting is not painful, horses should ambulate comfortably on the casted leg and tolerate having the contralateral limb briefly lifted for hoof cleaning. Any pain or reluctance to use the casted leg is a sign of a developing problem and should be investigated immediately. Often horses rapidly change from using the limb comfortably to being non-weight bearing on the limb. This may be due to cast breakage, breaking of the casted leg, or the development of a cast sore, among other things. The cast should be firmly palpated daily for signs of breakdown or cracking and the clinician should pay attention to the sound the horse makes when walking. Typically the cast begins to creak or crackle when cast failure and breakdown are imminent.

Cast sores are the most common complication in a cast and inevitably develop in the majority of cases. Sores commonly develop on the dorsal surface of the leg at the top of a cast, at the base of the fetlock, on the heel bulbs, and over any bony prominences on the leg (Figure 11.7). Sores can be mitigated by appropriately positioning the limb, adding protective padding or bandage material in known trouble spots, and ensuring the cast tape is applied with no wrinkles. Positioning the limb in a neutral weight-bearing or toe-touching/heel-elevated position results in the fewest cast sores and is most comfortable for the patient. Placing orthopedic felt at the top of the cast and over the heel bulbs adds a protective layer in those areas to reduce sores. Applying a layer of elastic tape without tension directly on the skin, as in Figure 1.5, not only helps to secure any bandage dressings and seal off an incision, but also acts as a second skin that protects against sores.

Developing or suspected problems should not be ignored and should be investigated immediately. Beyond physically examining the cast and leg, the clinician should consider radiographs to evaluate the position of the limb within the cast and if an abnormal position is contributing to discomfort. Occasionally, mild patient discomfort due to a slightly malpositioned cast can be addressed by adding or removing acrylic/epoxy on the cast bottom to relieve some pinching or rubbing. Unfortunately, these steps may not do enough or anything at all to improve patient comfort and continued wearing of the compromised cast will only contribute to the development of further problems. The most reliable way to address a cast problem is to remove the faulty cast and replace it with a new, properly positioned and applied cast. Even though this can add substantial cost to the care of the animal, removing a faulty cast can mean the difference between a successfully treated live patient and a catastrophic failure.

On rare occasion a cast may need to be applied to ensure limb stability with the need for access to the underlying limb for wound treatment, or the need for pressure relief over a certain area such as a pointed fracture end that may pierce the skin. In those instances a window may be cut in a cured cast using a cast saw to relieve pressure or allow access to a wound. If this is done for wound treatment, the removed cast material may be taped back in place to cover the wound following treatment (Figure 11.8).

(a) (b) (d)

(c)

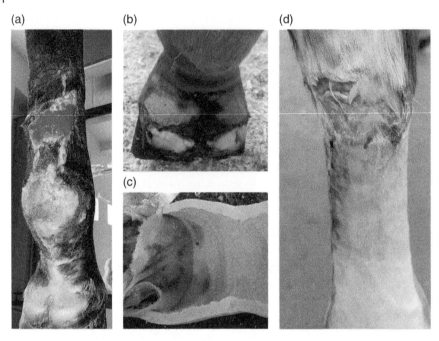

Figure 11.7 Appearance and location of common cast sores. (a) This patient is being treated for a complete superficial and deep digital flexor tendon laceration (notice the red granulation tissue) and has developed cast sores (pink areas) at the palmar aspect of its fetlock and on the heel bulbs, due to the lack of tendon support on the limb and subsequent malpositioning of the limb within the cast. (b) Cast sores developed on the heel bulbs of this patient within 24 hours of cast placement as a result of wrinkles in the cast material during cast application for wound management. The horse became non-weight bearing lame overnight and was instantly more comfortable once the cast was removed. (c) Notice the wrinkles on the inside of the cast, which caused the sores shown in (b). It is very easy for wrinkles to occur in this area of the cast due to the rapidly changing contour of the equine limb distal to the fetlock. This can be somewhat mitigated by using narrower cast tape for the initial layer and carefully wrapping the cast material during application. (d) This patient developed a cast sore on the dorsal aspect of the metacarpus at the top of a half limb cast. It resulted in full-thickness erosion of the skin in that area, which required additional bandaging and wound care following cast removal.

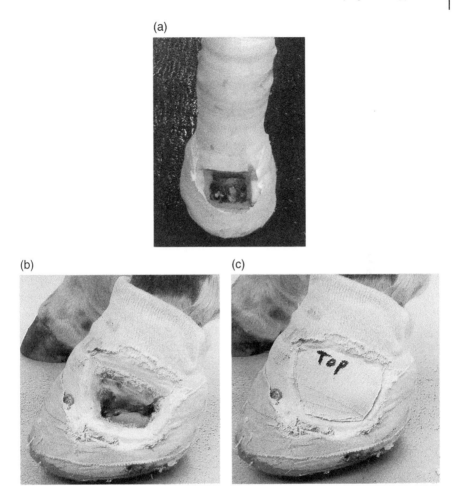

Figure 11.8 Examples of cast windowing. (a) Here a window has been removed from the dorsal aspect of a half limb cast over the hoof to allow wound treatment of an infected surgical site. (b) A window was cut in this foot cast to allow wound treatment over an area of hoof wall resection. (c) The removed portion of cast material in (b) was saved and labeled to allow it to be replaced in the cast window to be secured in place with elastic tape.

Cast Removal

While cast changes usually occur under general anesthesia due to the requirement to protect the still healing leg, final cast removal is usually performed with the horse standing and well sedated. The timing of cast removal is dictated by the nature of the injury and the clinician's assessment of healing. Frequently, horses are transitioned from a cast into a bandage for a period of days or weeks to manage the healing of any cast sores or additional wound healing that needs to take place.

Casts are removed through a process termed "bivalving" or "clam shelling," whereby two full-thickness cuts are made through the cast material at 180° from each other, most commonly on the medial and lateral aspects of the cast. The cast cuts can be done with an oscillating cast saw (Figure 11.9) or through the use of fetotomy wires strung through intravenous tubing that were placed at the time of cast application. Some clinicians prefer to bivalve the cast dorsally and palmarly/plantarly. Proponents of this latter approach claim that cast removal is easier because it eliminates limb flexion while prying apart the cast halves and does not require the clinician to reach around to the inside of the leg. However, this latter approach places the clinician directly in the striking/kicking zone should the patient react and increases the risk of damage to the flexor tendons should the cast saw cut too deeply.

Use of an oscillating cast saw takes practice to correctly, safely, and efficiently remove a cast. Clinicians should practice on a cadaver limb before using a saw on a live patient to avoid iatrogenic damage to the patient. Considerable care needs to be taken to feel for the change in resistance to ensure the clinician does not cut too deeply and harm the patient's skin or deeper structures. Cutting too deeply can severely injure vital structures such as a joint, tendon, or ligament. Though usually relatively benign, this can be catastrophic and a healthy dose of respect should be given to the cast saw at all times.

When using an oscillating saw the cut is not made by a longitudinal back-and-forth "sawing" motion. Instead, it is made by placing controlled pressure on the cast at the proximal aspect and allowing the vibration of the saw to cut the material from superficial to deep until a "give" can be felt as the cut runs fully through the cast material. Then the saw blade is lifted from the cut, moved distally 1–2 cm so that the blade overlaps the previous cut by less than 50%, and the process repeated. As the cut progresses to the full cast length, an assistant can place a broad, flat-head screwdriver in the gap of the cut and twist it by 90° to assess if the cast material has been fully cut. If the gap widens when the screwdriver is twisted then the clinician knows a full-thickness cut has occurred, but if the gap does not widen then the cut must carefully be redone until full-thickness transection has been achieved. Once the cast material is fully cut on both sides of the limb, cast

(a)

(b)

(c)

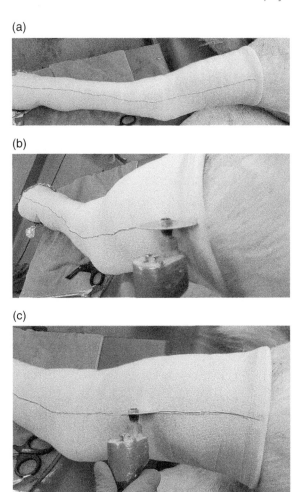

Figure 11.9   Use of an oscillating cast saw for cast removal. (a) A full rear limb cast is prepared for removal. When using a cast saw it is important to evenly split the cast into two halves. Drawing a line down the middle of the cast on both sides is helpful to ensure you do not get off track during the process. (b) The cut should begin at the top of the cast. The oscillating saw blade should be carefully pressed into the cast material. The operator should guard themselves against cutting too deeply and may brace their hand against the cast to assist in this (not shown). The image here illustrates the depth of the saw blade that has made a full-thickness cut. When this occurs the operator will notice a distinct change in resistance to the down pressure, at which point they should quickly lift the saw from the cut. (c) Once a full-thickness cut is made, the saw blade is moved distally approximately 30–50% of the width of the blade and again pressed into the cast material, feeling for the "give" indicating a full cut has been made. The blade should be maintained in alignment with the previous cuts to ensure each cut connects with the previous ones. This sequence is continued distally until the entire side of the cast has been cut.

(d)

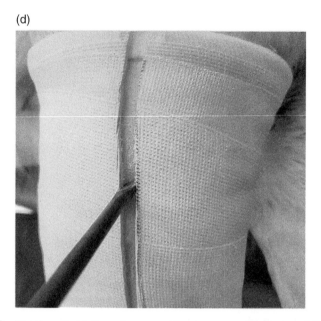

Figure 11.9 (Continued) (d) Once the cast cut has been completed, a broad, flat-head screwdriver is inserted with the width of the flat blade parallel with the cut. The screw driver is then rotated 90° (shown here) and the cast observed to be spread slightly. This indicates that a full-thickness cut has been made in that region. The screwdriver is moved distally several centimeters and the process repeated. If a full-thickness cut has not been made, then resistance will be felt and the cast material will not spread. The screwdriver can be moved proximally and distally slightly to twist and localize the area where the cast has not been fully cut. The cast saw is then carefully used make a deeper cut to release the cast material. Once completed, the process is repeated on the inside of the leg. Cast spreaders (not shown) can be inserted medially and laterally into the gap in the cast material, facilitated by the use of the screwdriver. The spreaders are squeezed to loosen the cast and assistants grasp the spread cast to further pry it loose. Bandage scissors should be readily available to assist in cutting the underlying layers to allow full cast removal.

spreaders are placed in the cut gap and used to spread the cast halves open. At this stage it is helpful to have an assistant ready with bandage scissors and two assistants present to grasp the cast halves and pry them open (Figure 11.10). Once all of the cast material, padding, and stockinette have been removed, the limb is cleansed, sutures removed, wounds treated, and a bandage is placed as dictated by the attending clinician.

(a)

(b)

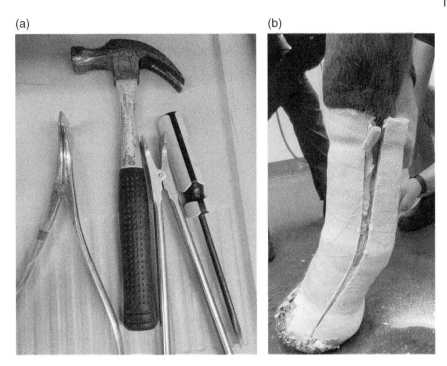

Figure 11.10   A half limb cast being removed in a standing patient and equipment needed for removal. (a) Two different styles of cast spreaders are shown as well as a large flat-head screwdriver used to facilitate introduction of the spreaders. The hammer can be used with a chisel (not pictured) to remove excessive acrylic from the cast prior to cutting with a cast saw. (b) Spreading of the cast just prior to removal. The individual to the right has inserted cast spreaders and the individual to the left is cutting the layers of stockinette and cast padding with bandage scissors. Notice how the cast has been cut evenly with roughly half dorsal and half palmar, creating two equal parts that can be easily removed. If the cuts are made too far dorsally or palmarly, the cast may still wrap around the leg and removal will not be possible.

Suggested Reading

Elce, Y. (2017). Bandaging and casting techniques. In: *Equine Wound Management*, 3e (ed. C. Theoret and J. Schumacher), 146–155. Ames, IA: Wiley.

Watts, A. and Fortier, L. (2020). Casting and transfixation casting techniques. In: *Nixon Equine Fracture Repair 2* (ed. A. Nixon), 188–206. Hoboken, NJ: Wiley.

12

Hoof and Phalangeal Casts

Wounds and trauma commonly occur to the hoof and phalanges of a horse. Occasionally, a surgery must be performed that weakens the integrity of the area. Management of third phalanx fractures and laminitis are other disorders where hoof capsule stability may be needed. Immobilization of these compromised structures facilitates the healing process, improves patient comfort, and can reduce impact on the owner by eliminating the need for frequent bandage changes. This chapter illustrates the process for applying a cast to each region.

Hoof Cast

Once the hoof capsule's integrity has been compromised, it must be supported until the damaged area has grown out. This may be accomplished by the application of a purpose-built shoe by a farrier. Often the damaged hoof needs more support than a shoe can provide and a hoof cast can be applied to provide that support (Figure 12.1 and 12.2). It may even be used to provide material for the farrier to secure a shoe using nails. In other instances a farrier is not readily available and a cast must be used to stabilize the hoof capsule until a farrier is able to apply a shoe.

Equine Bandaging, Splinting, and Casting Techniques, First Edition. J Dylan Lutter, Haileigh Avellar, and Jen Panzer.
© 2024 John Wiley & Sons, Inc. Published 2024 by John Wiley & Sons, Inc.
Companion website: www.wiley.com/go/lutter/1e

(a)

(b)

(c)

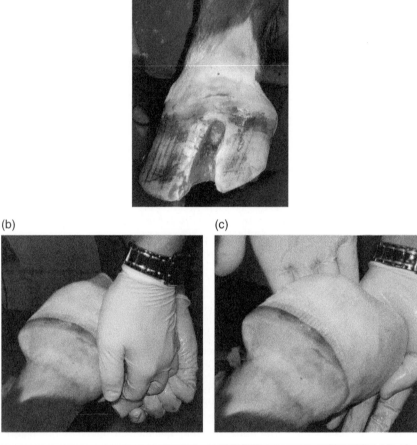

Figure 12.1 (a) A hoof wall resection has been performed on this hoof to remove a keratoma tumor. This subsequently compromised the hoof capsule integrity. (b) Cast tape is being applied around the hoof capsule, being careful not to encroach on the coronary band. Once the entire roll of cast tape is applied, the free edge is folded and smoothed flat on the solar surface of the hoof. (c) The finished hoof cast will immobilize the hoof capsule until the inflammation from surgery can subside and a farrier is available to apply a custom shoe. This cast was bandaged over to protect the wound and no hoof acrylic was applied to the bottom.

(a)

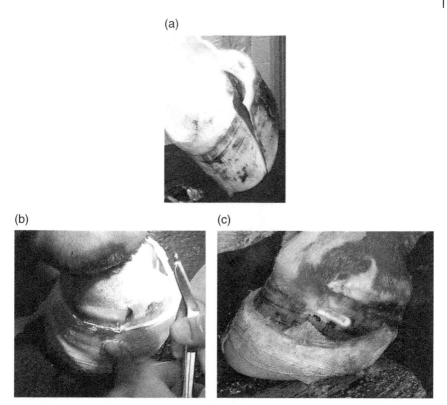

(b)   (c)

Figure 12.2   (a) This horse has lacerated its lateral hoof capsule and coronary band, nearly transecting the entire lateral quarter and heel. (b) Cast tape has been applied circumferentially to the hoof. Portions of the tape are being trimmed to remove pressure over the coronary band and heel bulbs. The wound will then be managed with a bandage. (c) The appearance of the healing wound after several weeks of stabilization and treatment, in preparation for application of a custom shoe.

Phalangeal Cast

Phalangeal casts, otherwise known as foot casts, enclose not only the hoof capsule but also the heel bulbs and pastern region of the horse. The materials needed for a phalangeal cast are illustrated in Figure 12.3 and listed in Table 12.1.

These casts are very useful to stabilize heel bulb and pastern lacerations (Figure 12.4). They also can be used to help manage pain in horses with laminitis (Figures 12.5–12.9) and may aid in stabilizing the hoof capsule prior to application of therapeutic shoes. Finally, some configurations of a third phalanx fracture that are being managed conservatively may not be adequately stabilized by just a hoof cast and require a phalangeal cast to improve patient comfort.

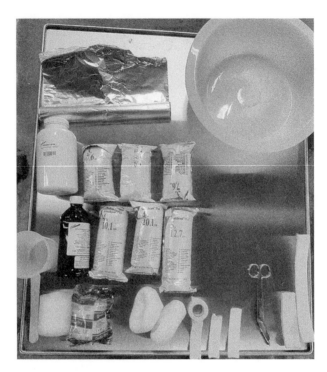

Figure 12.3 Materials to have on hand for a phalangeal cast.

Table 12.1 Supply list for a phalangeal cast.

Material needed	Number needed
Wound dressings as dictated by the wound	
Rolled stockinette – size dictated by patient size	1
Orthopedic felt, 1 in. wide strip	1 – long enough to encircle the pastern 1 – long enough to cover the heel bulbs
1 in. athletic tape	3 strips, to secure the felt
Cast padding	1 roll
Bandage scissors	1 pair
2 in. cast tape roll, optional	1
3 in. cast tape roll	1–3
4 in. cast tape roll	1
5 in. cast tape roll	1
Aluminum foil roll	Approx. 12–15 in. (30–38 cm) length
Acrylic powder and liquid (polymethlymethacrylate, PMMA)	1 bottle each
Mixing bowl and stir stick for acrylic	1 each
Bowl or bucket of warm water	1
Box of exam gloves	1

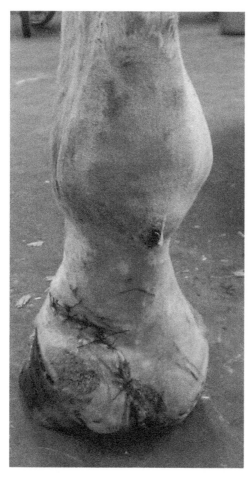

Figure 12.4 A common configuration of a heel bulb laceration that responds very well to management in a foot cast.

(a) (b)

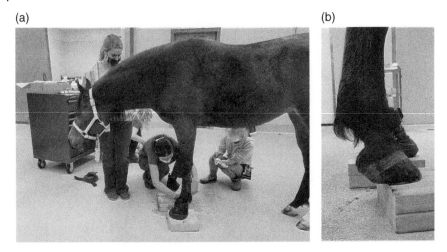

Figure 12.5 Application of a phalangeal cast in a standing patient. The patient is being managed for an acute on chronic instance of laminitis. In this case the clinician is working with a DVM/certified journeyman farrier to stabilize the laminitis in preparation for application of therapeutic shoes. Not every case of laminitis needs or responds to application of a foot cast. Some cases can worsen despite application of the cast. Use of a foot cast in this way should only be attempted through consultation with experienced individuals. (a) The hospital environment, sedation, horse handling, and patient positioning are vital components of a successful and safe cast application in a standing patient. Here a dedicated horse handler is standing on the same side as everyone involved. She is standing near to the head of the horse, facing the horse and the limb being cast, while grasping the horse's halter and closely observing the procedure. Her job is to anticipate and prevent (if possible) any movement of the horse, while being prepared to move the horse away from people should the horse react in an unsafe manner. The horse is adequately sedated with its head lowered, drooping eyes/ears, and is not reacting to its surroundings. Oversedation of the horse is particularly problematic for cast application because the patient becomes unsteady and is often unable to stand firmly in place during casting. The procedure is taking place in the center of a quiet, well-lit, spacious, uncluttered area so that there is room for all those involved to move safely. All individuals are focused on the procedure and are on the same side of the horse. All are squatting in a safe position and no one is kneeling. Kneeling is particularly dangerous because it places your legs in danger of being stomped on and slows your ability to stand/move should the horse move on top of you. The horse is positioned on wooden blocks to facilitate cast application. All four of its limbs are placed squarely underneath the horse in a normal standing position. A horse that is positioned with one or more limbs in an abnormal position is unstable/uncomfortable and is likely to move at some point during the procedure. Additionally, if the cast is being placed on the unnaturally placed leg, the cast locks that limb into an abnormal position that will contribute to the development of cast complications and detract from patient comfort. (b) It is important to precisely place the horse's feet on the wooden blocks. A sufficient amount of the heel should be left overhanging the edge of the block to allow the cast material to be sufficiently wrapped beneath the heels and lock them into place without destabilizing the horse's stance and making it feel unsteady. Often nerve blocks have been used to numb the foot for laceration repair, which may facilitate the horse's willingness to stand in this unnatural position. At most, the caudal 50% of the hoof should overhang freely, with roughly 30% overhang being a more typical stance. The contralateral limb should be firmly placed in the center of an equally sized wooden block to maintain the balance of the horse.

(a)
(b)
(c)

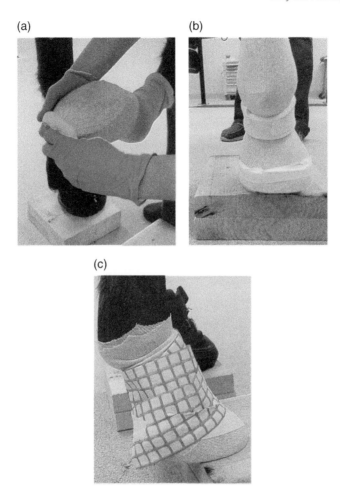

Figure 12.6 (a) To begin the casting procedure for the horse in Figure 12.5, any wound dressings are applied as dictated by the nature of the wound. Then the foot is picked up and the double-layer stockinette is rolled onto the limb approximately 4 in. (10 cm) proximal to the top of the cast. For this foot cast, the stockinette is rolled above the fetlock. The foot is then replaced on the block with the appropriate amount of overhang. (b) Following stockinette placement, the orthopedic felt is applied to the limb and secured with short strips of athletic tape. A circumferential 1–2 in. (2.5–5 cm) wide strip of ½ cm thick orthopedic felt is placed at the intended most proximal aspect of the cast and secured with tape. The heel bulbs are protected with another strip of similarly sized felt that covers just the heel portion and does not encircle the hoof. Some clinicians may prefer to fully encircle the coronary band with felt, while others may elect to omit felt at this location. (c) Then the cast padding is applied to the limb with the top edge neatly aligning with the top edge of the orthopedic felt, leaving roughly ½ in. (1 cm) of felt exposed to protect the limb. Here, Gore Procel cast padding has been applied. Note that this cast padding does not neatly conform to the leg and wrinkles or odd overlaps are to be expected. This does not seem to negatively impact the cast or cause problems. Note that the stockinette has been trimmed to extend just past the proximal extent of the cast. This trimmed edge should be folded over the cast material just prior to applying the final roll of cast tape and then covered with cast material for a neat and tidy cast.

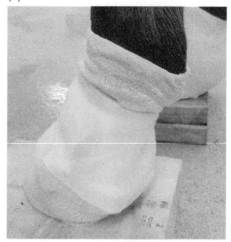

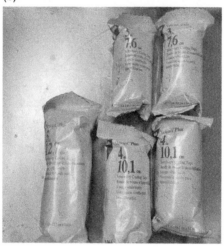

Figure 12.7 (a) The appearance of Delta-Dry cast padding for comparison to the Procel in Figure 12.6. Note how this material more easily conforms to the leg. (b) Three rolls of cast tape are typically used for application of a phalangeal cast, but it is a good idea to set out at least one additional roll of the most common size to use as a back-up. The width of the cast tape is important for the first layer of any cast, but particularly for a phalangeal cast because it is such a short cast being placed in an area with many contour changes. The narrowest cast tape available at the clinic should be chosen for the initial layer of the cast. This narrow tape conforms to the limb and does not tend to wrinkle easily. The authors have used 2 in., 3 in., and 4 in. cast tape for foot casts, but most often choose 3 in. because it conforms well and is of sufficient width to provide good coverage during application. If desired, the entire cast can be applied with 3 in. tape. The 2 in. tape tends to wrinkle less, but is not sufficiently wide to provide cast tape coverage without gaps forming that then need to be wrapped over. The 4 in. tape provides excellent coverage of the leg, but is too wide to conform to the foot without forming wrinkles during the initial layer of application. Generally, a wider roll of casting tape can be used after the initial roll is applied. This wider roll of tape provides better coverage over the limb and a more uniform surface to promote bonding of the cast material layers and subsequently a stronger cast. The 5 in. cast tape is reserved for the final roll used to cover the toe and sole of the horse's hoof.

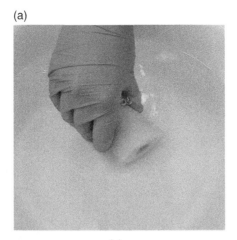

(a)

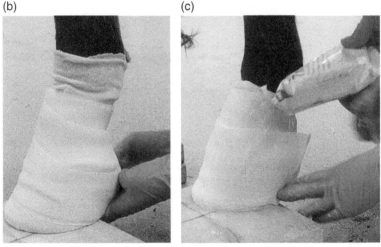

(b)   (c)

Figure 12.8 (a) Once the cast padding has been placed for application of a phalangeal cast in a standing patient, the first roll of cast tape is fully submerged in the warm water. The roll is held submerged until it ceases to produce bubbles and cast application promptly begins. The authors do not generally squeeze the cast material, but some clinicians may prefer to do this and some manufacturers may recommend doing so. (b) The initial roll is applied so that the top edge aligns with the top edge of the felt, leaving ½ in. (1 cm) of exposed felt. An initial circumferential wrap is then taken, similar to bandage application. The cast tape is applied to the limb with minimal tension and wrapped distally with approximately 50% overlap of the tape width. In the phalangeal cast, this will only be two or three wraps until the heels of the foot are encountered. Once the heel bulbs are encountered, the cast tape is wrapped beneath the heels onto the freely overhanging solar surface of the hoof. Wrapping is then continued dorsally over the coronary band and proximal hoof capsule, leaving the toe of the hoof exposed. Wrapping continues proximally, maintaining 50% overlap until the top edge of the cast is encountered. When one roll ends, the second roll should begin where it left off. The cast applicator should be particularly vigilant that there is appropriate cast tape overlap and that no wrinkles or dog ears are forming, especially on the initial layer of cast tape. If any occur during application, that wrap should be backed off and re-applied. Notice here that the stockinette has not yet been rolled down onto the cast material. (c) As subsequent rolls of cast tape are applied, it is common for the inner portions not to be fully wetted. If this occurs, water should be poured onto the cast tape as it is being applied. An opened cast tape wrapper is particularly useful as a water scoop. Notice here that the stockinette was rolled onto the cast and subsequently covered by the final roll of cast material.

(d)

(e)

(f)

(g)

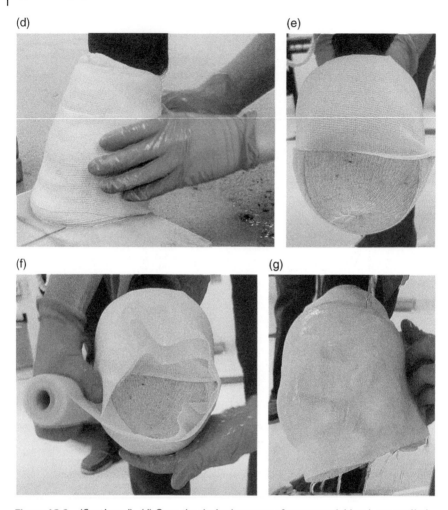

Figure 12.8 (Continued) (d) Once the desired amount of cast material has been applied, a minimum of five to six layers, the cast material is rubbed as it begins to set. This promotes bonding of the cast material layers and smooths the outer surface of the cast. As the cast material becomes hard, the rubbing can cease and the cast be given time to cure, typically an additional five minutes. (e) Once the cast has hardened to the point where it will not move, the limb can be picked up and positioned for the final layer of cast material to be applied. Notice the amount of cast coverage on the solar surface of the heels. The cast material is covering the palmar third of the frog sulci and fully covering the heels. It is important that this portion of the hoof is covered in this manner so that the foot is locked into place and the limb can be picked up without danger of the foot moving. (f) The 5 in. roll of cast tape is wetted and applied. Three complete wraps are taken around the hoof so that half of the cast tape width is secured on the hoof and half is left freely hanging. This free-hanging portion will be later conformed to the solar surface of the hoof. (g) After the three circumferential wraps, the cast tape is wrapped "freestyle" in a figure-eight or crisscrossing pattern so that the entire toe and solar surface of the hoof are covered with as much cast material as possible. If needed, more water can be applied during this process to fully wet the inner layers of the cast tape roll.

(a)　　　　　　　　　　　　　　　　(b)

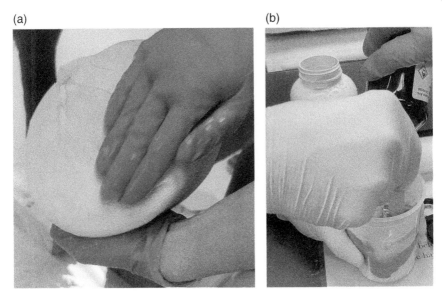

Figure 12.9 (a) Once the entire 5 in. roll of cast tape has been applied to the horse in Figure 12.8, the material is flattened and smoothed onto the sole of the hoof. It is continually rubbed and held into place until the cast has cured. At that point the foot can be set back onto the wooden block in preparation for the next step. (b) Once the cast has fully hardened, a protective layer for the solar surface must be applied. Without this layer the horse will quickly walk through the bottom of its cast. The authors prefer to use polymethyl methacrylate (PMMA) hoof acrylic, which is made of two parts, one powder and one liquid. Experience will help the clinician judge how much powder is needed to adequately cover the cast bottom. Somewhere between one and two cups of powder are commonly used. The liquid portion is then carefully mixed with the powder so that excess liquid is not introduced. If excess liquid is used, then additional powder can be sprinkled and mixed into the acrylic until the desired consistency is reached. It is important to wear gloves during the mixing and application of the acrylic as the material will firmly bond to the skin. It should also be noted that the aroma of the acrylic is quite strong, similar to that of a nail salon, so mixing in a well-ventilated area is helpful.

(c)

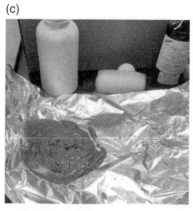

(d) (e)

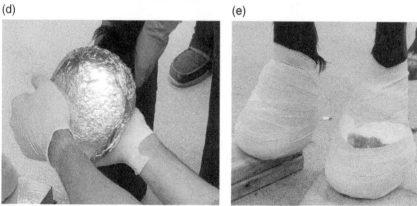

Figure 12.9 (Continued) (c) Acrylic that has been mixed to the correct consistency and poured onto a sheet of aluminum foil, just prior to application. This is a time-sensitive process as the acrylic hardens with an exothermic reaction. The acrylic should not be runny like cake batter and should be a thicker consistency, like brownie batter, so that it maintains some form when poured. It should not be so thick as to resemble cookie dough. If the acrylic is too runny, the clinician can either add a small sprinkle of powder and carefully mix it, or simply wait for the acrylic to begin to self-harden before applying. If the acrylic is too thick, due to a lack of liquid being added, then some may be added at this time, but mixing will be difficult as the foil is easily torn. If the acrylic is too thick because it has begun to fully cure, then it may need to be thrown away and the process started again. (d) Once the acrylic is fully mixed, of the proper consistency, and poured onto the foil, it is applied to the bottom of the cast and the foil wrapped around the sides of the cast to contain the acrylic. It is important that some of the acrylic be applied to the edge and distal sides to promote adherence of the acrylic to the cast. The cast applicator then uses their gloved hands to smooth and form the acrylic as it hardens. This can be a difficult and prolonged task if the acrylic was too runny when applied. Some clinicians prefer to apply the acrylic in a flat manner. If this is the case, the foot can be set down once the exothermic reaction has begun. Other clinicians prefer to mold a curved or domed bottom to the acrylic so as to facilitate break-over during ambulation, as is shown in this image. If this is the case, the limb must remain held until the acrylic has fully hardened. (e) Once the acrylic has fully cured, it should be covered with elastic tape to provide grip on the bottom of the cast. Some clinicians will also cut or grind a grip pattern into the bottom of the acrylic, but the authors have not found this necessary. Finally, the top of the cast is sealed with elastic tape to prevent intrusion of debris into the cast.

13

Bandage Casts

Wounds on the equine distal limb are a common occurrence in practice. Many times these wounds occur in an area of high motion that requires immobilization to prevent the dehiscence of a laceration repair or to provide the stability necessary to promote wound healing. These wounds typically require frequent care, which prevents the application of a cast (Figure 13.1). In these cases, the clinician has two options: immobilize the limb with a bandage/splint or apply cast material over the top of the bandage. The latter option can then be bivalved and the cast shells retained to use as a custom circumferential splint that can be re-used for subsequent bandages.

Materials required for a half limb bandage cast are listed in Table 13.1. The initial bandage cast application process is shown for a half limb in Figure 13.2 and the re-application of a bivalved bandage cast is shown for a carpal tube cast in Figure 13.3.

Equine Bandaging, Splinting, and Casting Techniques, First Edition. J Dylan Lutter, Haileigh Avellar, and Jen Panzer.
© 2024 John Wiley & Sons, Inc. Published 2024 by John Wiley & Sons, Inc.
Companion website: www.wiley.com/go/lutter/1e

(a) (b)

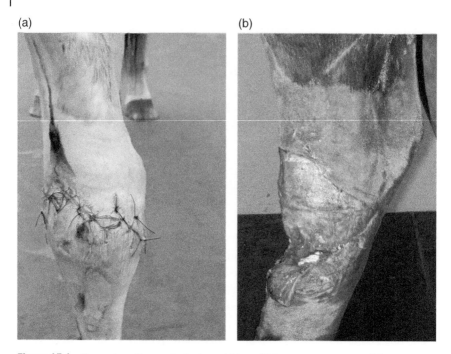

Figure 13.1 Examples of wounds that would benefit from management with a bandage cast. (a) A freshly repaired carpal laceration just prior to bandage cast application. (b) A tarsal degloving laceration on presentation prior to wound repair.

Table 13.1 Materials list for a half limb bandage cast application.

Material needed	Number needed
Cotton combine roll	1 roll, pre-packaged or self-cut to approx. 50 cm length
6 in. brown gauze	1 roll
4 in. cohesive bandage	1 roll
Elastic adhesive tape	1 roll
3 or 4 in. cast tape	2–3 rolls

(a)

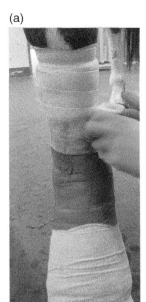

(b)

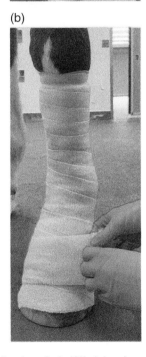

Figure 13.2 Process for application of a half limb bandage cast. (a) To begin, a standard bandage is placed routinely with appropriate wound dressings. The desired width of cast tape is fully wetted by submersion in warm water and then applied to the bandage. The cast tape begins at the top margin of the bandage, leaving approximately one finger's width of padding above the edge of the cast material. One wrap of the cast tape is taken and then wrapping continued distally with 50% overlap of the width of the cast tape. Here 3 in. cast tape is being applied at the discretion of the bandager, but 4 in. tape could easily have been used as well. (b) The cast tape is wrapped distally until the distal margin of the bandage is reached, being sure to leave a finger's width of padding distal to the edge of the cast material before wrapping is continued proximally while maintaining the 50% overlap.

(c) (d) (e)

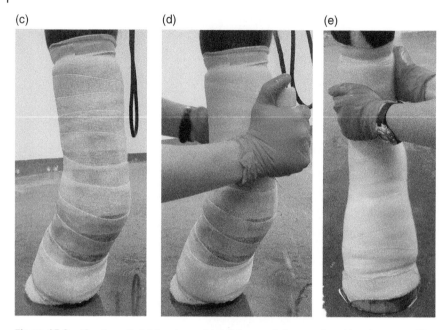

Figure 13.2 (Continued) (c) A palmar view of the partially completed bandage cast. The initial roll of cast material has run out after just two wraps distally and the bandager is awaiting the second roll of cast material. Notice that the distal margin of the bandage fully covers the soft tissues of the heel bulbs, protecting them from the cast material. (d) The second roll of cast tape is being applied. Here the bandager has chosen to begin this roll at the top of the cast. Alternatively, the roll could have been started on the distal aspect where the initial cast roll ran out. In this case, the decision to start the second roll at a different location will have minimal consequence as a single wrap of material will not create a large discrepancy in cast thickness. Cast tape is applied as previously described until a minimum of five to six layers of cast material have been applied. (e) After the final roll of cast tape has been applied, the cast material is rubbed to promote bonding of cast layers and to smooth the outer surface of the cast. It is important that the patient remain still until the cast resin has fully cured. At that point the cast may remain uncut until it is time for a bandage change. Alternatively, the cast may be bivalved and re-secured with inelastic tape to eliminate the need for cast cutting at a later time.

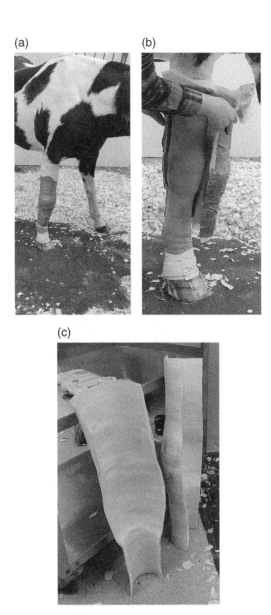

Figure 13.3 Process for re-application of a carpal tube bandage cast. (a) Here, a patient with a carpal laceration is prepared for a bandage cast change. Notice that the horse is well sedated and standing firmly on its legs. Patients do not always require sedation for a bandage change, but use of sedation to assist in restraint during the bandage change of a laceration in a high-motion area can reduce the risk of an unwanted step being taken by the patient with the cast removed. Also notice how the patient is positioned near the door in the stall with the clean shavings swept away from the limb for the bandage change. (b) The duct tape is cut on one side and the previously bivalved cast shell is removed. The bandager then quickly moves forward with the necessary steps to complete the bandage change and wound care. (c) During the bandage change an assistant removes the tape from the cast shell and checks the cast material for damage or cracks prior to placing the halves back in an easily reachable location.

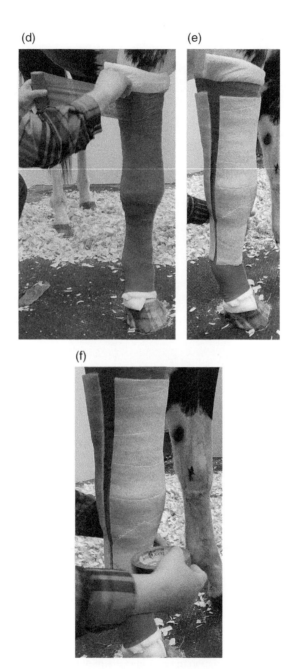

Figure 13.3 (Continued) (d) The final layers of the bandage are being applied. It is important that the bandager pays close attention to the contours of the bandage as materials are applied and tries to match the original bandage contour as closely as possible, to ensure the cast shells fit appropriately. (e) The cast shells are firmly pressed onto the leg. The bandage is assessed for any gaps or ill-fitting points. (f) The distal aspect of the cast is squeezed tightly together and secured with one to two wraps of inelastic tape. This is done intentionally before the top aspect to prevent distal slippage of the cast during tape application.

(g) (h) (i)

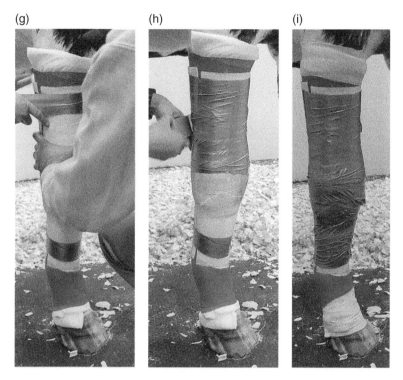

Figure 13.3 (Continued) (g) An assistant squeezes the cast halves closely together as the bandager tightly tapes the proximal aspect of the cast. (h) Inelastic tape is tightly wrapped distally with 50% overlap until the cast material is fully covered. (i) The completed carpal bandage cast, which can be kept in place until the next bandage change, typically in two to three days. If needed or desired this can be maintained for up to four to five days as long as the cast or bandage does not slip.

14

Half Limb Casts

Half limb casts are useful for stabilization of a wide variety of conditions. Often they are placed with the horse under general anesthesia following a surgical procedure such as an arthrodesis or fracture repair. While it is often preferential to use general anesthesia, these casts may be placed with the horse standing under sedation if the horse is amenable and the situation dictates. The standing application progresses best with an experienced clinician in charge and a well-coordinated team. Front limbs may simply be held by an assistant with the carpus flexed, but rear limbs are more challenging because the reciprocal apparatus requires simultaneous flexion of the fetlock, tarsus, and stifle when the limb is held up. This can be somewhat circumvented by holding the rear limb just off the ground in extension, possibly resting the toe of the hoof on a block. Some horses may tolerate extension of the limb caudally with an assistant supporting the tibia (and essentially the entire hind quarter of the horse).

A final creative maneuver that may be used to facilitate casting a limb in a standing horse is to unroll a roll of 3 in. or 4 in. cast tape and fold it accordion style with the help of an assistant, similar to what is shown in Figure 8.1b, so that the length of the folded cast material is roughly 1.5–2 times the intended length of the half limb cast. The horse is then stood on the middle of the folded cast tape in a normal weight-bearing position and the remaining length of material folded up onto the dorsal and palmar/plantar aspects of the leg. Multiple assistants are typically required to hold the folded cast tape smoothly onto the leg while the main cast applicator begins wrapping the initial roll of wetted cast material to secure everything in place. Additional water is applied during the wrapping to ensure that all of the cast material is sufficiently wetted. This approach requires that the horse is able to bear weight on the leg. It can be quite tricky to correctly apply the cast and requires multiple assistants. All of this increases the risk of developing

Equine Bandaging, Splinting, and Casting Techniques, First Edition. J Dylan Lutter, Haileigh Avellar, and Jen Panzer.
© 2024 John Wiley & Sons, Inc. Published 2024 by John Wiley & Sons, Inc.
Companion website: www.wiley.com/go/lutter/1e

casting complications. As such, it is easy to see why it is preferential to place a half limb cast using general anesthesia. Materials required for a half limb cast are illustrated in Figure 14.1 and listed in Table 14.1.

This chapter demonstrates half limb cast application, first, in the anesthetized horse (Figures 14.2 & 14.3) and then in the standing, sedated horse (Figure 14.4). The authors recommend that standing half limb cast application not be undertaken until the clinician is comfortable with the procedure on an anesthetized horse. Finally, cast removal in the standing, sedated patient is discussed (Figure 14.5).

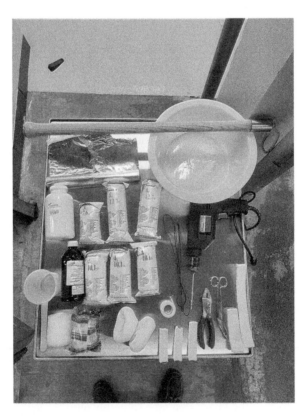

Figure 14.1 Materials to have on hand for a half limb cast.

Table 14.1 Supply list for a half limb cast.

Material needed	Number needed
Wound dressings as dictated by the wound	
Rolled stockinette – size dictated by patient size	1 roll
Orthopedic felt, 1 in. wide strip	1 long enough to encircle the proximal metacarpus/metatarsus
	1 long enough to cover the heel bulbs
1 in. athletic tape	3 strips, to secure the felt
Cast padding	1–2 rolls
Bandage scissors	1 pair
Electric drill and 3/16 in. or 4.5 mm drill bit	1
Malleable wire or fetotomy wire	18–24 in. (45–60 cm) length
Slip joint pliers	1 pair
Wire cutters	1 pair
3 in. cast tape roll – optional	1
4 in. cast tape roll	3–4
5 in. cast tape roll	1–2
Aluminum foil roll	Approx. 12–15 in. (30–38 cm) length
Acrylic powder and liquid (polymethlymethacrylate, PMMA)	1 bottle each
Mixing bowl and stir stick for hoof acrylic	1 each
Bowl or bucket of warm water	1
Box of exam gloves	1

Anesthetized Half Limb Cast Application

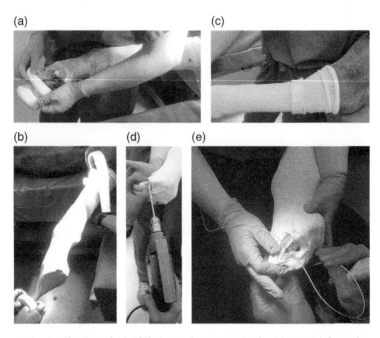

Figure 14.2 Application of a half limb cast in an anesthetized horse. (a) Once the affected limb's procedure is complete, the wounds/incision are dressed as indicated. The hoof is cleaned and trimmed if necessary, which was not done for this procedure. If the clinician desires, an antiseptic drying solution such as tincture of iodine or Kopertox is applied to the frog sulci to prevent the development of thrush within the cast. This was not performed in the patient pictured. Then, a double layer of stockinette of the appropriate size is applied to the limb. In this case, 4 in. stockinette is being applied. (b) After the first layer is rolled on, ending at least 3–4 in. (7.5–10 cm) proximal to the intended top of the cast, the second half of the stockinette is twisted once and rolled onto the limb. Notice that while this is happening an assistant is measuring the circumference of the proximal metatarsus just distal to the tarsometatarsal joint in order to cut the orthopedic felt to the correct length. (c) The 1–2 in. (2.5–5 cm) wide strip of orthopedic felt is applied circumferentially at the proximal aspect of the metatarsus. The head of the lateral splint bone serves as a good landmark for placement of the felt. It is important that the ends of the felt appose each other and do not overlap so that a pressure point is not created. Notice in the picture the slight overlap of the felt ends. This was corrected prior to the next step. On occasion, the contour of the leg prevents the felt from staying in place and it tends to slip distally. Because of this, some clinicians prefer to secure the felt temporarily to the skin using a penetrating towel clamp in addition to the tape. The clamp is removed after the initial roll of cast tape has been applied. (d) Next, small holes are cut in the stockinette medially and laterally at the widest part of the foot. A hole is drilled in each exposed hoof wall starting at the outer margin of the white line, angling abaxially, being careful not to encroach on the sensitive laminae. However, it is important to drill at a sufficient angle so that good-quality hoof capsule is penetrated to secure the subsequent wire placement. Pay attention so that the stockinette does not become caught in the spinning drill bit and become entangled. (e) Wire is threaded through the hoof wall holes, creating a loop on the solar surface.

(f)   (g)

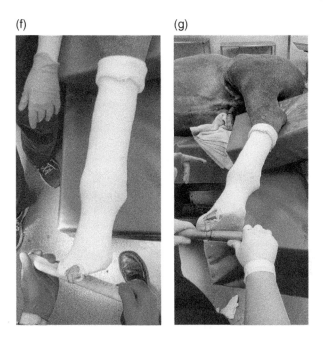

Figure 14.2 (Continued) (f) A handle is secured to the bottom of the foot by the loop as the wire is tightened. Here a cut section of twitch handle is being used, but often an entire twitch or other wooden handle is selected. The handle is used by one assistant to align the phalanges and maintain the foot in a neutral weight-bearing position. Another assistant should be available, standing near the abdomen, to secure the proximal portion of the limb. In the front limbs this person stands facing cranially and grasps the cranial aspect of the carpus or distal radius in order to maintain the carpus in extension for the duration of the casting procedure. In the rear limbs this assistant places proximal and caudal pressure on the patella to maintain the limb in a locked, standing position. Notice that the plantar aspect of the handle is pulling away from the heels. This is because the wire holes were drilled too far dorsally in this patient to adequately secure the handle. However, this is a minor issue as the handle is still sufficiently secured to maintain the position of the foot. Also notice that the proximal aspect of the stockinette has been folded distally on top of the orthopedic felt. It was folded to help secure the stockinette and prevent it from slipping distally following cast placement. Normally this is not done until after the first layer of cast material has been applied to provide a more secure point. (g) It is important that the limb be maintained in a neutral standing position with alignment of the bony column. This is relatively easy in the front limb by simply maintaining full carpal extension. In the hind limb this is more difficult. Special attention should be paid to placing the limb in a neutral position so that a line can be drawn from the coxofemoral joint distally through the center of the tarsus and fetlock and finally the palmar half of the foot. The assistant holding the limb should pay close attention to ensure that the limb is not being abducted or adducted and that they main the foot in neutral. A good guideline for a horse in lateral recumbency is to compare the hoof sole to the sternum of the horse and maintain the sole parallel to the sternum. If the limb is judged to be too far cranial or caudal, the entire limb should be picked up, moved, and placed in the correct location. The limb pictured here is in reasonable alignment, but could be moved slightly caudally to improve if the clinician desired.

(a)

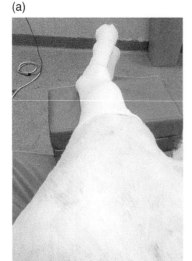

(b)

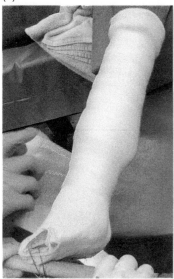

Figure 14.3 (a) A different perspective of hind limb positioning on another patient. Notice how the hind limb is in a normal weight-bearing position with the joints aligned as previously described. The handle has not yet been placed. It is helpful to recheck limb alignment after handle placement to ensure nothing has shifted. (b) Cast padding is applied to the limb with just enough tension to remove wrinkles beginning proximally, even with the top margin of the felt, and wrapping distally with 50% width overlap until the heel bulbs are covered. Typically, one roll of padding is sufficient for a half limb cast. Use of additional cast padding risks creating too much space between the limb and the cast, which would then allow limb movement inside the cast. Notice here that the clinician has elected to not place orthopedic felt over the heel bulbs. This is not customary, but it is up to each clinician to decide which materials to apply to which areas.

(c)

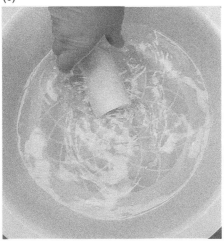

(d)

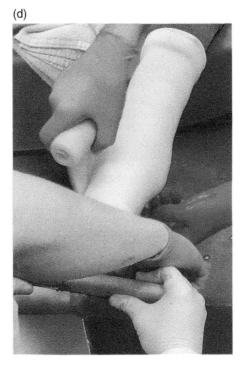

Figure 14.3 (Continued) (c) The initial cast tape roll is opened and submerged in warm water. It is important only to open one roll at a time, as exposure to humid room air can cause the water-activated resin to set prematurely. The widest tape that will smoothly conform to the limb without creating wrinkles should be used. Clinicians may elect to use 3 in. cast tape as the initial layer, but the authors have found that 4 in. tape can also be applied with similar ease and avoidance of wrinkles. (d) The cast tape is applied at the proximal margin, leaving roughly ½ in. (1 cm) of felt exposed to protect the skin from abrasion by the cast material. This initial layer is wrapped with minimal tension, progressing distally with 50% overlap. At this time, the cast material handler should be instructed to submerge the next roll of cast material to allow sufficient time for it to become wetted. The cast applicator should proceed quickly, while also paying close attention that the cast material is being applied smoothly and correctly.

(e)

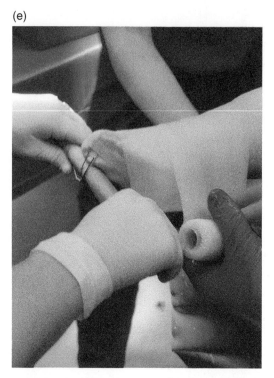

Figure 14.3 (Continued) (e) When the heel bulbs are encountered, special care is taken to wrap at least 50% of the tape width (or more) over the heels and covering the solar surface of the foot. This ensures that the foot is locked into place once the cast material cures. The cast tape then continues to be wrapped back proximally while maintaining the 50% overlap. Wrinkles are most likely to occur in this location because of the rapid changes in limb contour. Creative wrapping patterns can be used to try to avoid wrinkles while also moving the tape proximally and ensuring overlap of each subsequent wrap to avoid gaps. If wrinkles occur, the clinician should not be afraid to reverse course by one or two wraps to correct the wrinkle. If the wrinkle is noticed too late and several wraps have been applied, then an assistant can pinch the wrinkle to form a neat "dog ear" and carefully fold it over while holding it in place until it can be covered.

(f) (g)

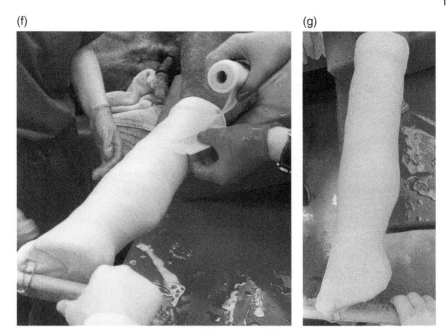

Figure 14.3 (Continued) (f) Once the end of a cast tape roll has been reached, the next roll should begin where the previous one ended. In this image the initial cast tape roll ended near the top of the cast and a second roll is being started. The applicator is being careful to wrap in the same direction as the first roll. The cast tape continues to be applied in this manner until at least five to six layers of cast material have been applied. Often the authors will use four 4 in. rolls and one 5 in. roll of cast tape during this process. Alternatively, you may use one 3 in., three 4 in. rolls, and one 5 in. roll. (g) The appearance and positioning of the cast after all intended cast rolls have been applied. Once the cast has cured, the wires in the hoof wall will be cut and removed. At this point, the cast is fully immobilizing the distal limb. The toe is still exposed and able to transfer forces to the limb. The remaining steps will be to fully enclose the foot and protect the cast from wearing through the bottom as the horse walks.

Standing Half Limb Cast Application

Application of a cast with the patient standing (Figure 14.4), under sedation, may be elected if circumstances preclude cast application under general anesthesia. Factors such as systemic illness, anesthetic risk, concurrent wounds or injuries, patient temperament, financial constraints, personnel, facilities, and time all need to be factored in to the decision to apply the cast in a standing patient. While excellent casts can be applied in this manner, there is an increased risk of cast complications due to limb positioning or movement as well as safety considerations for the people assisting with the procedure. Not every patient or situation will be amenable to the standing procedure. Clinicians should be familiar with and proficient in cast application in the anesthetized patient before attempting to apply a cast in the standing patient.

The materials necessary for standing cast application are the same as those for when the patient is anesthetized, except that the twitch handle is replaced with a wooden block or blocks for the patient to stand on. The clinician must decide, based on the injury at hand, if the limb should be positioned in a normal weight-bearing position or if the patient should be placed in a toe-touching stance. If a normal stance is chosen it is often best also to have the contralateral limb placed on a block to evenly distribute the weight and increase patient comfort during the procedure, as shown in Figure 12.5. If the toe-touching stance is elected the clinician must decide if the limb is to be held up by an assistant for the entire procedure or if the limb can be rested on a block in the desired position. Hind limbs, because of the reciprocal apparatus, can be especially challenging. Chapter 12 demonstrates cast application for a standing, normally positioned front limb and should be referred to for additional descriptions of patient positioning for that procedure. Figure 14.4 demonstrates cast application in a hind limb with the limb positioned in a toe-touching stance using a technique where the limb is pulled forward and the horse's toe is rested on a wooden block. This approach requires two additional assistants: one dedicated to maintaining the position of the limb and one dedicated to ensuring the hoof remains positioned on the block and the dorsal cortices of the digits and metatarsus remain aligned.

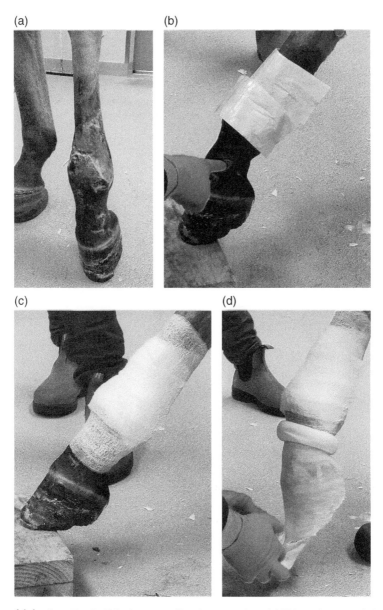

Figure 14.4 Standing half limb cast application procedure. (a) This patient was being managed for a severe laceration in the fetlock region that involved the fetlock joint. A cast was elected to promote wound healing after the joint was sealed and the soft tissue infection resolved. Standing application was elected due to client finances and the docile temperament of the patient. (b) Non-adherent pads are applied after the wound and leg are cleaned. Notice how the toe of the foot is placed on the block with the toe supported and the heels hanging freely off the edge. There should be sufficient contact so that the patient can bear enough weight to align the dorsal cortices of the metatarsus and the digits. This patient is being allowed to rest its leg until application of the cast material begins. (c) Woven gauze is applied to the limb without tension to secure the pads in place and act as an absorbent material for wound exudate. (d) A double-layered stockinette is applied to the limb as an assistant lifts the limb. Because the limb must be lifted, both layers are rolled over the hoof before completing the application to the limb.

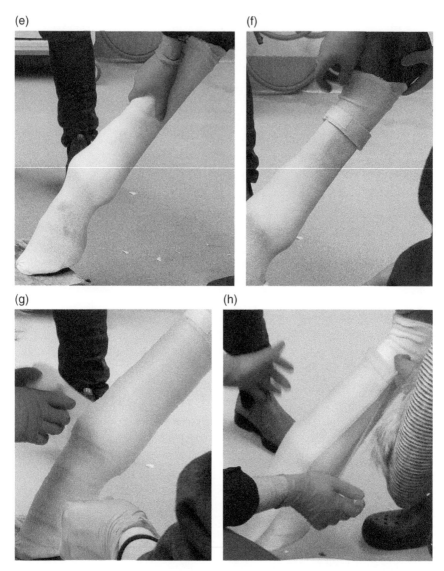

(e) (f) (g) (h)

Figure 14.4 (Continued) (e) The limb is replaced on the block. The material has been pre-measured to extend roughly a hand's width proximal to the intended top of the cast. (f) A 1 inch wide strip of orthopedic felt is placed at the proximal aspect of the metatarsus. It is identified by palpation of the heads of the second and fourth metatarsal bones. The felt is placed so the ends appose each other, do not overlap, and are secured in place by white athletic tape. (g) Cast padding is applied without tension to the limb from the proximal metatarsus distally to cover the heel bulbs. (h) Here an alternative approach to cast material application is shown. This is only useful for standing applications. It requires additional assistants to secure the cast tape during the application of subsequent material, which can be difficult and may increase the risk of wrinkles forming in the cast material. If the application is successful, the entire hoof and distal limb will be locked in place. To perform this method, a 4 inch wide roll of cast tape is unrolled and folded accordion style so that it is roughly double the intended length of the cast. The middle of this length is identified, the horse stood on the tape at that location, and each end carefully folded proximally to lie on the dorsal and plantar surfaces of the limb.

(i)

(j)

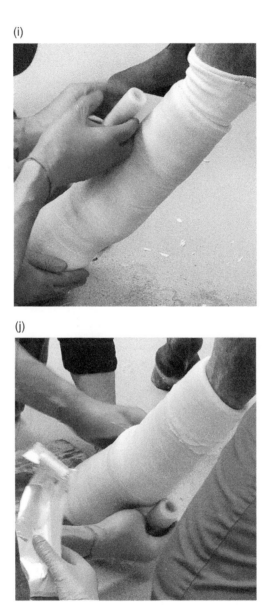

Figure 14.4 (Continued) (i) Cast material is applied to the limb with the top edge aligning with the top of the felt. For the initial roll, 3 or 4 inch wide tape may be chosen with subsequent rolls typically being of the 4 inch variety. Wrapping continues distally with 50% overlap with careful attention being paid to changes in contour of the limb and the formation of wrinkles or dog-ears. (j) When the heel bulbs are reached the cast tape is wrapped beneath them to cover the freely overhanging portion of the hoof and wrapping is continued proximally. The stockinette should be folded down after the first or second layer of cast material so that it is incorporated into the cast. Subsequent rolls of cast material should begin where the previous rolls end.

(k)

(l)

(m)

(n)

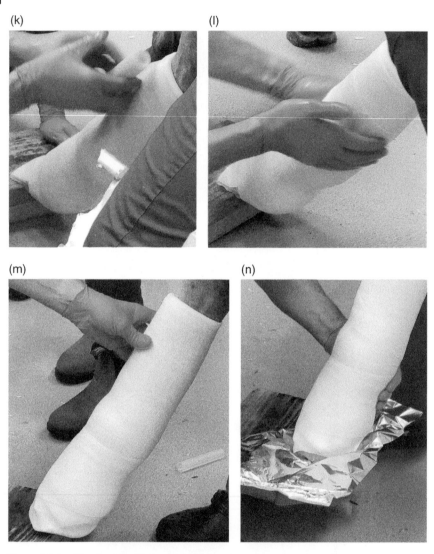

Figure 14.4 (Continued) (k) Care should be taken when the top of the cast is encountered to ensure that the cast tape edges align neatly. Cast tape application should be continued until at least six layers of cast material have been applied. More may be applied at the senior clinician's discretion. (l) Next, the cast should be gently rubbed with open palms until the resin begins to harden to promote bonding of the cast tape layers. (m) If clinicians elect to place the casted limb in the toe-touching position they plan for a wedge of cast material to be applied to the heels to increase the ground contact surface of the cast. Refer to Figure 14.3 to review this technique. Shown here is the cast at the end of the procedure with cast material fully cured. (n) After the cast has hardened, acrylic is applied to the bottom of the cast and held in place with aluminum foil.

(o)   (p)

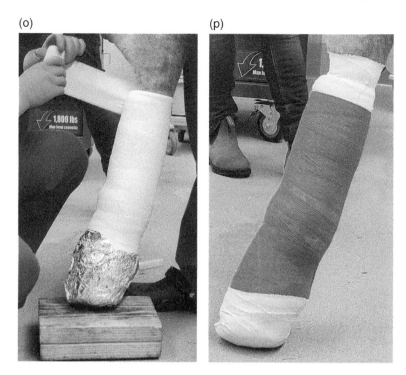

Figure 14.4 (Continued) (o) The foil is folded around the cast and the limb replaced on the block while the acrylic hardens. This creates a flat surface that increases the ground contact of the cast. This may make some patients feel more secure while standing on the cast but does little to facilitate ambulation. While the acrylic cures, elastic tape is applied to the top of the cast without tension, half on the cast and half on the haired skin to seal it. (p) Elastic tape is applied over the acrylic to increase the friction with the floor and reduce slipping. Shown here is the completed cast. Cohesive bandage material has been applied to this cast to keep the underlying cast clean while the patient is trailered to the referring veterinarian's clinic for continued care and observation.

Standing Cast Removal

Half-limb casts may be removed while the horse is standing (Figure 14.5), under sedation, once the need for the cast has resolved or the time for a cast change has arrived. The choice between standing removal or removal under general anesthesia is dependent on the initial injury and the extent of healing, both of which dictate the need to replace the cast, as well as on the temperament of the horse and financial constraints of the client. It is important prior to beginning the procedure that the horse be adequately sedated and not easily roused. Horses that are easily excitable by external stimulation may benefit from ear plugs or even blindfolding. If these techniques are employed it is imperative that extra care be taken to ensure human safety.

(a)

(b)

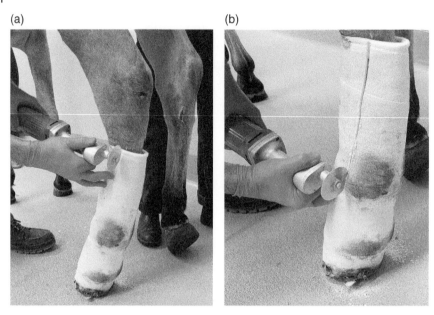

Figure 14.5 Standing cast removal of a half limb cast using a cast saw. This patient presented for a standing cast change after being managed at the referring veterinarian's clinic for five weeks for the severe dorsal fetlock laceration seen in Figure 14.4. Notice the contralateral limb support in the form of a wooden clog glued to the hoof and supported with a hoof cast. (a) To begin the cast removal the cast saw is held in two hands with the dominant hand holding the saw close to the blade. Notice that the clinician is supporting the saw by placing two fingers of his dominant hand against the cast to support and guide the blade as it is pressed into the cast material. The initial cut begins at the proximal edge of the cast and straight lateral to medial pressure is applied until a give in resistance is felt. The clinician must maintain careful control of the cast saw to immediately lift it once this change is sensed to avoid cutting the patient. (b) The saw blade is moved distally roughly 50% of the blade width, again carefully pressed into the cast, and quickly lifted from the cut once the resistance changes. This process is continued distally in a straight line until the bottom of the cast is encountered such that the cast will be divided into approximately equal dorsal and plantar halves. Not shown is the use of a wide blade screwdriver to spread the cast and ensure a full-thickness cut has been made. This concept is discussed in Chapter 11 and demonstrated in Figure 11.9d.

(c) (d) (e)

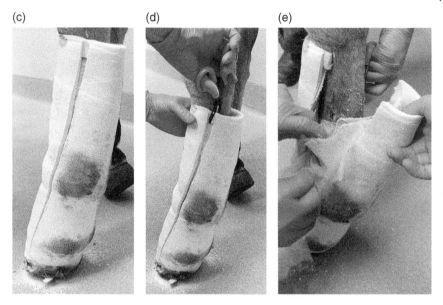

Figure 14.5 (Continued) (c) Once a full-thickness, full-length cut has been made, the cutting process is repeated for the medial aspect of the cast. Notice the gap that has begun to form without spreaders, indicating a successful cut. (d) Either simultaneously with or subsequent to the second cut an assistant uses scissors to cut the orthopedic felt, cast padding, and stockinette to facilitate cast removal. (e) Next, each half of the cast is firmly grasped by an assistant and the halves spread open. If needed, cast spreaders (Figure 11.10) may be used to facilitate the initial spreading of the halves, but these quickly become extraneous as the gap widens. An additional assistant uses bandage scissors to continue cutting the cast padding and stockinette.

(f)

(h)

(g)

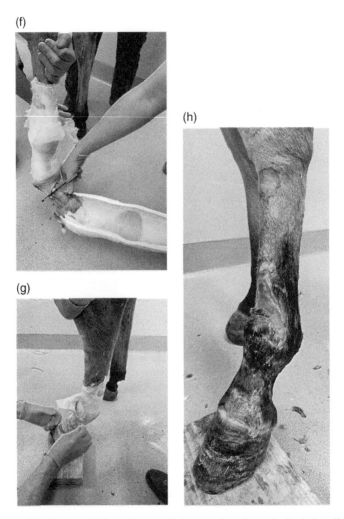

Figure 14.5 (Continued) (f) Once the cast halves are free from the limb the clinician picks up the leg for removal of any additional cast-related material. (g) The limb is placed in a standing position, in this case on a block, and any remaining bandage material is removed. The limb and any wounds are cleansed with surgical scrub before proceeding to any subsequently planned procedures. (h) Shown here is the appearance of the limb after cleansing. There is minimal evidence of casting complications despite the relatively long duration this cast was in place, save for a minor partial-thickness cast sore caused by pressure of the cast on the dorsal aspect of the proximal metatarsus. This wound is now ready for the granulation tissue to be trimmed. In some cases it may be appropriate to fit the leg with a bandage and splint for additional protection but less rigid immobilization. Rarely in a case like this are the tissues strong enough to be managed by only a bandage. In this case, an additional cast was applied to the limb following the trimming and dressing of the wound.

15

Full Limb Casts

Full limb casts are much less commonly applied and the principles are the same as for half limb casts. While the application principles are the same, full limb casts require more material (Figure 15.1 and Table 15.1), have more locations that require orthopedic felt, and drastically affect the horse's ability to use its limb, which makes limb positioning during cast application even more vital. The reader is referred to Chapters 11 and 14 for a more thorough discussion of cast application principles. The figures in this chapter give the context for full limb casts.

It should be noted that full limb cast application is not without risk to the horse. A cast with its proximal margin ending too distally in the diaphysis of a long bone (radius or tibia) brings with it the risk of concentrating stress at that location and fracturing the bone. Additionally, there is a risk of peroneus tertius rupture when a full rear limb cast is applied due to the reciprocal apparatus of the rear limb and the stresses that structure experiences during ambulation.

The most common reason for placing a full limb cast in general practice would be to immobilize the limb as a way to facilitate wound management or protect a laceration repair that extends over the carpus or tarsus. Often this will be applied in a tube cast or bandage cast configuration in a standing horse, but it may be configured to enclose the foot. True full limb casts may be more common in specialty practice to help protect a proximal limb fracture repair or other surgical site during anesthetic recovery and the post-operative period. A full limb cast may also be considered in an emergency situation for fracture stabilization prior to referral if the clinician feels that splinting will inadequately protect the fracture during transportation.

Clinicians should target the application of at least six layers of cast material, but should plan to use more for specific areas of reinforcement in regions of high stress. The widest cast tape should be used to increase cast layer bonding and

Equine Bandaging, Splinting, and Casting Techniques, First Edition. J Dylan Lutter, Haileigh Avellar, and Jen Panzer.
© 2024 John Wiley & Sons, Inc. Published 2024 by John Wiley & Sons, Inc.
Companion website: www.wiley.com/go/lutter/1e

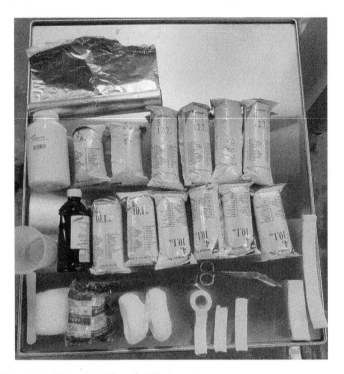

Figure 15.1 Materials needed for a full limb cast.

strength. Typically, 12 rolls of 4 in. or 5 in. cast tape are needed, but at least an additional 3–6 rolls should be available prior to beginning the application process to ensure that the entire limb is sufficiently covered with enough available for reinforcement.

Full limb casts should extend from the foot proximally to terminate just distal to the elbow or stifle joint (Figure 15.2). Strips of orthopedic felt should be placed circumferentially at the proximal margin of the cast and over the heel bulbs. Additional rings or "doughnuts" of felt should be placed over the accessory carpal bone, medially and laterally on the distal radial metaphysis/physis, over the medial/lateral malleoli of the tibia, and on the calcanean tuberosity. Since cast material is weakest in compression, areas that may sustain bending forces are prone to breaking or cracking. Additional cast material should be applied over the carpus and tarsus to strengthen these areas.

During application, particular attention should be given to the positioning of the leg in a normal weight-bearing position with the carpus/stifle locked in extension. The position of the phalanges can be changed by manipulating the foot and can be placed either in a neutral position with the sole parallel to the

Table 15.1 Supply list for a full limb cast.

Material needed	Number needed
Wound dressings as dictated by the wound	
Rolled stockinette – size dictated by patient size	1 roll
Orthopedic felt, 1–2 in. wide strip	1 long enough to encircle the proximal radius or tibia
	1 long enough to cover the heel bulbs
	3–4 doughnuts/rings of felt as needed to protect bony prominences
1 in. athletic tape	Strips as needed to secure the felt
Cast padding	3–5 rolls
Bandage scissors	1 pair
Electric drill and 3/16 in. or 4.5 mm drill bit	1
Malleable wire or fetotomy wire	18–24 in. (45–60 cm) length
Slip joint pliers	1 pair
Wire cutters	1 pair
3 in. cast tape roll – optional	1
4 in. or 5 in. cast tape roll	10–14 used; up to 18 available
Aluminum foil roll	Approx. 12–15 in. (30–38 cm) length
Acrylic powder and liquid (polymethlymethacrylate, PMMA)	1 bottle each
Mixing bowl and stir stick for hoof acrylic	1 each
Bowl or bucket of warm water	1
Box of exam gloves	1

sternum/floor or with alignment of the dorsal cortices (Figure 15.3). The authors prefer the former option, as it facilitates ambulation and increases patient comfort. If the cast is placed with the horse under general anesthesia, then clinicians should plan an assisted recovery with ropes on the head, tail, and possibly the casted limb. Recovery in a sling or pool is also an option, but is limited to facilities that are fully staffed and have clinicians experienced with these procedures. Once the horse is standing, clinicians should also plan to use a rope distally near the foot to help the horse advance the leg while walking.

(a) (b)

(c)

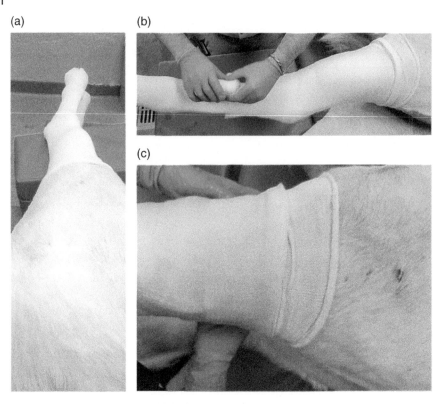

Figure 15.2 Application of a full limb cast in the hind limb of an anesthetized horse. (a) Once any wounds or surgical sites have been dressed, stockinette is applied to at least 4 in. proximal to the intended top of the cast. Orthopedic felt is applied at the level of the proximal cast margin, the heel bulbs, and any bony prominences. Then the limb is positioned to be in a normal weight-bearing position with the proximal joint locked in extension. The phalanges are positioned as described in Chapter 14, either in a neutral weight-bearing position or with the use of a heel wedge. (b) Cast padding is applied by starting at the proximal margin of the felt and wrapping distally with 50% width overlap. New rolls of padding should be started where the previous rolls run out and ended distally at the level of the heel bulbs. One layer of padding is sufficient, as additional rolls risk the cast being too loose fitting and allow excessive limb motion within the cast. (c) The initial roll of 4 in. or 5 in. cast material is submerged and fully wetted before starting application with the proximal edge being placed on the proximal strip of orthopedic felt, being sure to leave approximately ½ in. (1 cm) of felt exposed to protect the limb. At this time the subsequent roll of cast material should be submerged to ensure it is fully wetted.

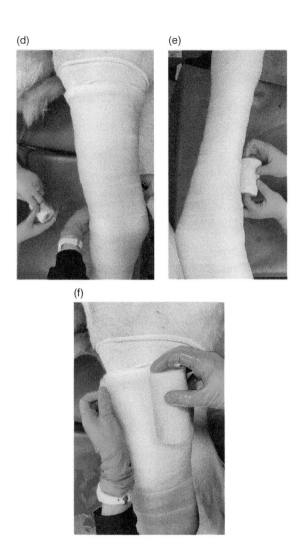

Figure 15.2 (Continued) (d) The cast tape is wrapped distally with 50% width overlap. An assistant stands at the ready with the next roll of cast material. Each subsequent roll should begin where the previous one ended to ensure an even-thickness application of the entire cast. In areas of bending or compression stress points, additional cast material wraps can be taken and the overlap width percentage increased to provide reinforcement. (e) Cast tape application continues distally, returning to 50% width overlap and being careful that only enough tension is applied to minimize wrinkles during the initial layer. Tension on the tape can be increased slightly with each subsequent layer of cast material. (f) Because of the large size of a full limb cast and the time it takes to apply the cast material, there is a real risk that each layer of cast material will begin to cure before the next layer can be applied. To mitigate this risk a second cast applicator may begin applying cast material once the initial cast layer has reached the level of the tarsus (or carpus if front limb). It is crucial that the cast tape be wrapped in the same direction as the previous rolls to ensure that cast application will continue smoothly, without wrinkles, and without interference between the cast applicators. The introduction of this second applicator brings with it additional complexity because at least one and possibly two additional assistants should be assigned to this second applicator, and the addition of a second applicator inherently brings the potential for more errors to be made. Nevertheless, if the team is sufficiently staffed and experienced this approach can greatly speed the process of full limb cast application and result in a well-bonded, stronger cast.

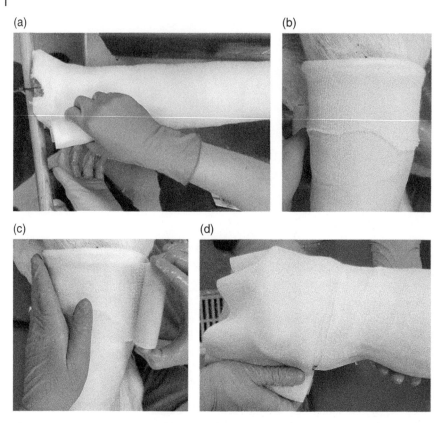

Figure 15.3 (a) Continuing the application of a full limb cast from Figure 15.2, once the heel bulbs are encountered the heels are locked into place by ensuring that one or two wraps cover the solar surface. This image shows the foot being stabilized by the use of a twitch handle with the heel bulbs in the process of being wrapped. The subsequent wrap will reach beneath the solar surface and the twitch handle before continuing proximally. (b) After the initial or second layer of cast material is applied, the stockinette can be folded down over the top of the cast to secure it in place. (c) The folded stockinette is covered during the process of cast tape application, with special attention paid to keeping the proximal margin of cast tape distal to the proximal margin of the orthopedic felt. Cast tape application continues until at least six layers of cast material cover the entire limb. (d) Once the cast has cured, the handle and wire can be removed and the foot covered by the application of a final 5 in. roll of cast material as described in previous chapters. The applicator ensures they cover the solar surface and toe as many times as possible with cast material. Any freely hanging cast material is folded over and held flattened to the solar surface until it is cured.

(e)

(f)   (g)

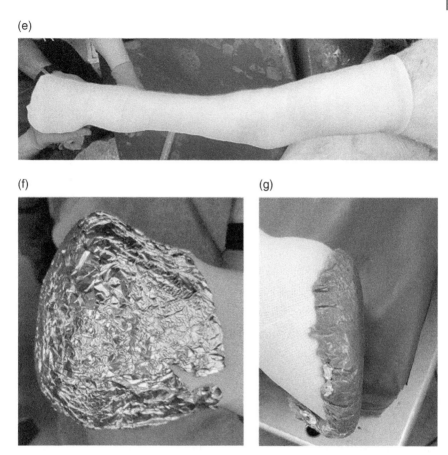

Figure 15.3 (Continued) (e) The appearance of the completed full rear limb cast with the foot enclosed. It is now ready for the application of hoof acrylic or epoxy to the solar surface. (f) The cast material is covered with hoof acrylic, which is then shaped and held in place until cured. Refer to Chapters 12 and 14 for more thorough descriptions of the acrylic application process. (g) The hoof acrylic has fully cured and the aluminum foil has been removed to show how the acrylic has been molded around the edges of the cast to help secure it to the cast. It is ready to be covered by elastic tape to reduce the slipperiness of the surface.

Index

Note: Page numbers referring to figures should be *italics* and those referring to tables in **bold.**

Equine Bandaging, Splinting, and Casting Techniques, First Edition. J Dylan Lutter,
Haileigh Avellar, and Jen Panzer.
© 2024 John Wiley & Sons, Inc. Published 2024 by John Wiley & Sons, Inc.
Companion website: www.wiley.com/go/lutter/1e